Realist Trials and Systematic Reviews

This book draws a line under the debate between realist evaluators and advocates of randomised controlled trials. Drawing on philosophical argument and practical examples, Bonell and colleagues show that realist trials and evidence syntheses can provide scientific evidence of effectiveness that is useful for decision-making. Realist trials cannot answer every evaluation question, but where randomisation is possible, such trials can be used to show whether an intervention works, and how its effects are shaped by the context in which it's delivered. Drawing on their extensive experience of conducting trials and systematic reviews of complex public health interventions, the authors show convincingly how the strengths of realist and experimental approaches can be combined. This is a book I'll be recommending to colleagues and postgraduate students interested in the philosophical underpinnings or the practical design of evaluation studies.

Peter Craig, Professor of Public Health Evaluation, University of Glasgow

The authors of this timely and readable book on approaches to evaluating complex interventions have thought hard about communicating difficult ideas. In straightforward language, ten chapters take us step by step through the history and arguments, using clear examples from their own work. The book doesn't shy away from controversy – the place of trials in realist evaluation, what a realist systematic review looks like – and one of its strengths is that it is framed as a proposition rather than as a prescription. Readers will welcome it as a primer that makes sense of a daunting field and covers a greater range and depth of knowledge than its brevity would suggest. I'll be recommending it as a first read for colleagues and students who want to evaluate complex interventions.

David Osrin, Professor of Global Health, UCL Institute for Global Health, UK

To anyone who has been involved in the long-running debate about different approaches to evaluation, this book comes as a huge relief. It takes a dispassionate, balanced and accessible look at the opposing sides: 'positivist' trials and systematic reviews versus 'realist' forms of evaluation. Chris Bonell and his co-authors show how the best of both approaches can be brought together to address the constant challenge of shaping public policies that are genuinely health- and welfare-promoting. We need to know what kinds of intervention work, but we also need to understand something about for whom and under what conditions which interventions are most appropriate. *Realist Trials and Systematic Reviews* should be required reading for all who work in the evaluation field, and policy-makers would benefit from more than a dip into its laudable commonsense.

Ann Oakley, Professor of Sociology and Social Policy Social Research
Institute University College London

Realist Trials and Systematic Reviews

Rigorous, Useful Evidence to Inform Health Policy

Chris Bonell
London School of Hygiene & Tropical Medicine

G. J. Melendez-Torres
University of Exeter

Emily Warren
London School of Hygiene & Tropical Medicine

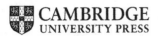

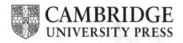

Shaftesbury Road, Cambridge CB2 8EA, United Kingdom

One Liberty Plaza, 20th Floor, New York, NY 10006, USA

477 Williamstown Road, Port Melbourne, VIC 3207, Australia

314–321, 3rd Floor, Plot 3, Splendor Forum, Jasola District Centre,
New Delhi – 110025, India

103 Penang Road, #05–06/07, Visioncrest Commercial, Singapore 238467

Cambridge University Press is part of Cambridge University Press & Assessment,
a department of the University of Cambridge.

We share the University's mission to contribute to society through the pursuit of
education, learning and research at the highest international levels of excellence.

www.cambridge.org
Information on this title: www.cambridge.org/9781009456609

DOI: 10.1017/9781009456616

First published 2024

A catalogue record for this publication is available from the British Library

A Cataloging-in-Publication data record for this book is available from the Library of Congress

ISBN 978-1-009-45660-9 Paperback

Contents

Figures

Tables

Boxes

Acknowledgements

We would like to thank the following people who co-authored papers with us which have greatly informed this book: Elizabeth Allen, Richard Amlôt, Laura Bear, Vashti Berry, Annah Chollet, Simon Cousens, Steve Cummins, Val Curtis, Calum Davey, Diana Elbourne, Rhiannon Evans, Caroline Farmer, Adam Fletcher, Ann Hagell, James Hargreaves, Richard Hayes, Farah Jamal, Fraizer Kiff, Betty Kirkwood, Theo Lorenc, Nick Mays, Martin McKee, Rebecca Meiksin, Susan Michie, Graham Moore, Laurence Moore, Matt Morton, Simon Murphy, Norren Orr, Mark Petticrew, Ruth Ponsford, Sidnei Priolo Filho, Audrey Prost, Stephen Reicher, Emma Rigby, Andrew Rizzo, David Ross, James Rubin, Nichola Shackleton, Naomi Shaw, Bruce Taylor, Russell Viner, Robert West, Lucy Yardley and Honor Young.

We would also like to thank others with whom we have written who have helped us develop our ideas: Sara Bragg, Rona Campbell, Andrew Copas, Matt Dodd, Angela Harden, Lauren Herlitz, Rosa Legood, Ann Oakley, Kathryn Oliver, Charles Opondo, Sara Paparini, Miranda Perry, Stephen Scott, Annik Sorhaindo, Vicki Strange, Jo Sturgess, Neisha Sundaram, Tara Tancred, Nerissa Tilouche, Meg Wiggins and Obioha Chukwunyere Ukoumunn.

We would also like to thank the following people, discussions with whom have helped clarify our thinking: Joanna Busza, Tim Colbourn, Brian Flay, Frances Gardner, Ford Hickson, Paul Montgomery, David Osrin, Jeremy Segrott, James Thomas, Nick Tilley and Peter Weatherburn.

Most of the evaluations and systematic reviews that we have conducted and which have informed this book have been funded by the Public Health Research Programme of the National Institute for Health Research. We are grateful for this funding. The views expressed in this book are those of the authors and do not necessarily reflect those of the National Institute for Health Research, the National Health Service or the Department of Health and Social Care for England.

Chapter 1

Introduction

1.1 Evaluating Complex Health Interventions

This book is about understanding the impacts of health interventions. By interventions, we mean actions that are purposefully taken to bring about specific, intended benefits. These actions could include implementing policies, modifying services, launching new social programmes or finding other new ways of working with patients or citizens. We are interested in *complex* health interventions. These are interventions that are more than just giving a pill or doing a particular medical or surgical procedure. They involve multiple components that interact with each other and with the context in which they are delivered.[1] Our own scientific research focuses on public health interventions, which aim to prevent disease or promote population health. Most of the public health challenges that we face today, such as preventing violence, obesity, infectious diseases or mental illness, are complex. They require interventions to address multiple influences on health operating at the level of individuals, communities and whole societies. These interventions might involve communicating health messages, providing people with support, persuading people to change their behaviour or changing the environments in which people live to make healthier decisions easier.

These interventions are complex firstly because they have multiple components that interact with each other.[2] The harder it is to say what the 'active ingredient' of an intervention is, the more likely it is to be a complex intervention.[3] Consider the 'Intervention with Microfinance for AIDS and Gender Equity' intervention. This aimed to reduce HIV infections and gender-based violence among poor women and their family members in rural South Africa. It did so by providing workshops which educated the women about HIV and gender, empowering the women by enabling them to work together to lead campaigns in their communities on issues of importance to them and providing the women with small loans to start small businesses and ease their poverty.[4] The intervention developers believed that all these components would work together so that women had the knowledge, motivation and life circumstances necessary to reduce their own and their family members' risk of HIV and gender-based violence. In other words, they hypothesised that the impact of the overall intervention would be greater than the sum of its parts.[5] But it is not only public health interventions like these that can be complex. Healthcare interventions can also be complex, even when they may not appear to be. The care that patients receive is not usually just limited to a single pill or procedure. It involves various activities which interact with each other. For example, interventions to remind pregnant women to take up a glucose tolerance test for gestational diabetes can include 'cues to action' for providers, different types of reminders for pregnant women and the provision of resources to facilitate women's ability to use a glucose tolerance test.[6]

Secondly, a clue that interventions could be complex is if they work differently across different contexts, that is with different populations or in different settings.[2][7] How interventions are delivered and the impact they have will depend on local factors, such as whether they are supported by local policies, whether potential implementation partners are ready to deliver them, whether they reach local people and whether they meet the needs of those they are meant to benefit.[8] The local capacity to implement an intervention and the local capacity to benefit from a complex intervention will vary. Consider the example of using youth service interventions as a way to prevent teenage pregnancies. The intervention might involve a youth worker mentoring young people, giving young people additional education on academic and life skills and facilitating group activities to build self-esteem and raise aspirations. Interventions of this sort have been found to reduce teenage pregnancy rates in New York City but not in other parts of the USA.[9][10] Some of us evaluated a government-led pilot programme to implement this sort of intervention in England and found that it actually *increased* the rate of teenage pregnancy.[11] Various factors might explain these differences in impact across different contexts. In England, the youth work was sometimes provided as an alternative rather than a complement to normal schooling so the students referred into it might have felt like their involvement labelled them as failures. The youth work itself sometimes was delivered with low fidelity so it did not match up to what was intended. In New York City, the intervention was delivered to all young people living in areas of poverty. However, in England the intervention was targeted to particular young people whom teachers or social workers judged as at particularly high risk of pregnancy. The intervention might have increased the rate of pregnancy in this English context by bringing together the most at-risk young people, possibly leading to more sex without contraception.[12] A useful way to think about an intervention is that it is a disruption to an existing social system. By social system, we mean the places, environments and community values and practices that shape what we believe and how we behave. The pre-existing features of this system will shape how the intervention is delivered. And different social systems will be 'disrupted' in different ways by the same sort of intervention, with implications for local impacts.[13] This book will provide an approach to evaluation which rigorously assesses the outcomes of interventions and how these vary between contexts.

1.2 Why Evaluation is Important

In this book, we argue that the evaluation of complex health interventions and the use of this evidence to inform policy are critically important but currently are not achieving their full potential. The reason why evaluation is important is because it is usually not obvious what impacts complex interventions have. Interventions might bring about lots of benefits or they might do nothing, waste money or even harm people. Even if they are beneficial in some contexts, interventions may not work everywhere, as the above example of youth work and teenage pregnancies demonstrates. Interventions are always delivered with good intentions, but it is often not obvious to those delivering or receiving interventions what impacts (if any) they have had. The impacts might be too subtle to be noticed. We don't need evaluations to tell us that parachutes work but most interventions do not generate such dramatic outcomes as do parachutes. It can also be difficult to distinguish intervention impacts from other changes happening at the same time.

One problem is 'regression to the mean'. This occurs, for example, when clients or places receive an intervention for the very reason that, at that moment, they are at heightened risk of some adverse outcome. Their risk naturally fluctuates up and down over time, and it goes down to a lower level at about the same time as they received the intervention without this being a result of the intervention. For example, you might seek an HIV safer sex counselling intervention when you are concerned about your current risk of HIV. You might have gone on holiday and had more sex than usual or used protection less than you normally would. Your level of risk will probably dip back down independently of any impact of the counselling.[14]

Another problem is distinguishing the effects of an intervention on a population from the broader trends affecting that population. There might be 'maturational trends' (people changing as they get older) or 'secular trends' (people being affected by long-term historical changes). Because of these trends, it can be hard for those delivering or receiving an intervention to separate the 'signal' (intervention effects) from the 'noise' (other trends or events). This issue can also challenge evaluators, a subject we will turn to in Chapter 2.

A particularly important role for evaluation is to detect harms. No one wants to continue to deliver an intervention that causes harms. But, like intervention benefits, these may not always be obvious. 'First do no harm' is an ethical requirement that ranks higher even than doing good.[15] Although it is easy to imagine how medicines or surgery could inadvertently cause patients harm, it is harder to imagine that interventions such as education, social support or environmental improvements might cause harm. Unfortunately, however, lots of evidence indicates that this can sometimes happen.[12] As well as the example of youth work and teenage pregnancy described in the previous section, another classic example is that of the Cambridge-Somerville social work intervention. This involved providing a broad set of social work interventions, such as counselling and free places on summer camps, for at-risk boys in New England, USA, in the 1930s. Those who received the intervention were found to experience higher rates of criminal activity, alcoholism and mental illness later in life.[12] Because interventions are interruptions to complex social systems, it is plausible that unintended effects can occur, some of which might be harmful.[16] The assessment of harms has been a neglected topic in evaluations of public health interventions,[17] other than for a few topics such as suicide prevention and illicit drug interventions.[18][19] But interest in the potentially harmful effects of public health intervention has increased recently and researchers have tried to define different categories of harm.[12][17] One way to do this is to distinguish between 'paradoxical effects' (the intervention making worse the very thing it is trying to make better) and 'harmful externalities' (the interventions bringing about harms in completely different areas).[20]

Interventions often aim to reduce health inequalities. These are avoidable, unnecessary and unfair differences between groups in health status and outcomes. These may arise as a result of the unequal distribution of resources or as a result of discrimination or other unequal access to rights. Minoritised and racialised groups experience worse health outcomes across a range of conditions. Women experience disproportionate impacts from intimate partner violence. People experiencing poverty are less able to access health services. Interventions may often aim to reduce health inequalities, but some will actually increase health inequalities, benefiting the health of the advantaged more than the disadvantaged even if the health of no individuals is directly harmed by an intervention. When interventions disproportionately benefit people who already have better health, we call this an 'equity harm'.[17] Conversely, interventions that decrease gaps between groups in health status can be said to create 'equity benefits'. Certain types of interventions, such as mass media interventions, are known for being more likely to create equity harms because only those already most able to take up mass media messages do so.[21] Our book will identify approaches that ensure that evaluation can rigorously assess not only whether interventions achieve their intended effects but also whether they generate any harmful effects.

But evaluation is expensive, complicated and time-consuming. We cannot evaluate every intervention all of the time to make sure that it is benefiting and not harming those it aims to help. We need to decide when to evaluate interventions and when not to bother. If the intervention has dramatic, obvious effects, an evaluation is not needed unless there are concerns of possible harmful externalities. If an intervention is cheap, easy to deliver, acceptable and there is minimal risk of harm, it may also not be worth evaluating.[22][23] It may also not be worth evaluating an intervention if it is delivered as a one-off with no plans to repeat it over time or in different places. But an intervention might be worth evaluating if its expected impacts are subtle; if it is costly, difficult or controversial to deliver; if it has the potential for harmful effects; and if it will be delivered in more than one time or place.

A single evaluation study is unlikely to provide a definitive guide to whether an intervention is a potentially useful approach to use across contexts. The results of a single study may be biased by limitations in the methods used or the biases of those leading the evaluation. A single evaluation undertaken at a single point in time and in a single place is unlikely to provide evidence that will allow us to decide where else and for whom else the intervention should be delivered. So we usually need multiple studies to better understand intervention effects. The results of these individual studies need to be critically appraised and their results summarised in what are known as 'systematic reviews'. In Chapter 2, we describe conventional approaches to evaluation and systematic reviews, and some of the limitations with these conventional approaches.

1.3 The Value of Evidence in Informing Policy

Evaluation and the use of evidence to inform policy have a long history. Authors such as Donald Campbell, Robert Merton and Karl Popper, writing in the mid-twentieth century, argued that we need experiments to inform and assess government policies.[24–26] Popper termed this 'piecemeal social engineering', meaning incremental changes to policies or services which are then evaluated to assess whether they have the intended impacts or whether they have caused unintended harms. At this time, there were only a few examples of large-scale evaluations in areas such as agriculture, education, medicine and social work (including the Cambridge-Somerville study). Most policy decisions were made on the basis of tradition, political ideology or simply the views of those in charge. The last of these is well illustrated by the statement that 'the gentleman [sic] in Whitehall really does know better what is good for people than the people know themselves'[27] (p. 317).

Popper saw evaluation and the basing of policy on evidence of impact as a way to resolve tensions between conservative, liberal and socialist ideologies that were playing out between the eighteenth and twentieth centuries.[25] Conservatives thought that societies should stick with traditional ways since these were tried and tested, representing the collective wisdom of previous generations. Liberals wanted new policies to improve social conditions and promote individuals' welfare and rights. Socialists demanded or anticipated radical changes to how the economy was run to make societies fairer. Popper argued that radical policy change was often grounded in theories about society for which there was no evidence. These policies could bring about unintended harms (such as tyranny, violence and mass starvation). The speed and scale of these policy changes could leave insufficient time for evaluation or improvement. Popper, as well as Campbell and Merton, recommended that social policies should focus on gradual change and empirical evaluation of their effects. Karl Popper proposed piecemeal social engineering informed by experimentation.[25] Robert Merton argued for the importance of developing scientific theory informed by evidence to guide policy.[26] Donald Campbell coined the term 'the experimenting society' as a way to think of how policy change could progress based on careful trial and error.[28] Popper viewed social democracy as the form of government which could gradually address the inequalities generated by capitalism, ensuring that citizens received education, health and welfare, and were entitled to civil and worker rights.[25] In liberal democracies, the idea that policy should be based on evidence started to become more popular in the 1960s and became really influential from the 1990s. During this period, when centrist and centre-left governments ran many countries, evidence-informed policy came to be associated with a 'technocratic, Third Way' approach, summed up in Tony Blair's phrase 'what matters is what works'.[29]

Some critics argue that the use of evaluation and other research evidence to inform policy and practice is merely part of the apparatus through which the state and experts control service providers and citizens.[30] They argue that using evidence in this way narrows policymaking to a series of expert-led technocratic assessments squeezing out democratic consideration of values and priorities. Evidence, it is argued, can be a way to obscure the political way in which the powerful decide what counts as a 'problem' or a plausible 'solution'.[31] Quantitative evidence is regarded by some critics as particularly problematic because, it is argued, it tends to prioritise precision (in estimating what factors cause or what interventions affect health outcomes) over depth (in terms of analysing the broader social structures which bring these problems about).[32][33] It is argued that the use of insufficiently 'upstream' analyses then informs the use of insufficiently upstream interventions so that the deeper causes of health inequalities remain unexamined and unchallenged.[32][33] We disagree with such analyses; the use of evidence from evaluations and other research need not bring about undemocratic and de-politicised decision-making. There is no inevitable trade-off between statistical precision and depth of analysis.[32] Use of quantitative evidence need not preclude the assessment of how deeper social forces contribute to health inequalities or the impacts of interventions addressing these forces.[34][35] In this book, we offer recommendations for how evaluation can contribute to evidence-based policymaking in more useful ways than has been achieved to date.

1.4 The Strengths and Current Limitations of Randomised Controlled Trials and Systematic Reviews

We strongly support the use of randomised controlled trials, (or trials for short), where possible, to assess the impacts of complex health interventions. We also strongly support the use of systematic reviews to collate evidence from multiple studies and using this to inform policy decisions. We believe that trials and systematic reviews offer the most scientifically rigorous means of determining the impacts of interventions. Trials produce the least biased statistical estimate of how much better are the outcomes of people who are allocated to receive an intervention compared to those who are allocated not to receive this. Systematic reviews collate evidence from various studies to provide the most comprehensive answer to the question of whether or not an intervention 'works'. In Chapter 2, we explain why this is so.

However, while we believe that randomised trials and systematic reviews, when done well, are very scientifically rigorous as methods, we argue in this book that they are often not scientific enough in their overall orientation, that is what questions they ask and what evidence is used for. They generally focus on questions of *if* and *how much* interventions work, and generally do not focus enough on understanding *how* interventions work and *for whom* or *where* they work best. This is a critical gap in the evaluation of complex health interventions because, by definition, these interventions work via complex mechanisms, which also interact with local context, to generate different impacts in different places or populations. Because of the failure to consider context and mechanism in meaningful ways, evaluators cannot provide policymakers or practitioners with the evidence that they need to decide if the intervention in question may be beneficial beyond the context of the original evaluation. In Chapter 3, we argue that this seriously limits the usefulness of evaluation evidence in informing policy.

Some people argue that the reason trials are not very useful is that they try to apply methods from the natural sciences to understand how the social world works. Complex interventions involve interactions between people, with people deciding how to change their actions based on their understanding and experience of an intervention. Critics argue that trials (and science more generally) are just not appropriate to understanding this messy and nuanced social world.[36] We disagree with this position. Instead, we argue in Chapter 3 that the evaluation of complex interventions actually needs to become more, not less, scientific. Currently, evaluation, including trials, is generally limited to being a sophisticated form of intervention monitoring. Evaluations *describe* the impacts of an intervention statistically and use this as a basis for 'accrediting' interventions as effective or not (in Tony Blair's terms 'what works'[29]). Instead, we argue, trials need to contribute to testing and refining scientific theories about how and for whom interventions work.

In Chapter 3, we draw on ideas from 'realist' evaluation methods to develop a method by which trials can become more scientific. We call our method 'realist trials'. We describe this method in detail in chapters 4, 5 and 6. In chapters 7 and 8, we consider how the method can also be applied to improving systematic reviews. We call this approach 'realist systematic reviews'. In Chapter 9, we consider how our methods can help make evidence more useful in informing policy decisions. In Chapter 10, we consider how our methods can be used to test and refine scientific theories, which might then in turn be used to inform interventions and policy in the longer term. Our ideas are controversial and some researchers disagree with our approach.[37][38] But we hope to present arguments and evidence to show that ours is the right approach.

Why Are Trials and Systematic Reviews Necessary but Currently Insufficient to Inform Health Policy?

In Chapter 1, we considered why evaluation and using evidence to inform policy is so important. We also made two assertions. The first is that randomised controlled trials and systematic reviews offer the most scientifically rigorous methods of generating and summarising evidence about the effects of interventions. The second is that randomised trials and systematic reviews are currently not scientific enough in their orientation, which makes them much less useful than they might be in informing policy. But we did not provide any justification for either of these assertions. In this chapter, we consider both of these in more detail and hopefully offer some convincing arguments about both.

2.1 How Do Randomised Trials Work?

Randomised controlled trials (or 'trials' for short) have been used for decades to evaluate not only biomedical interventions but also complex interventions in fields such as economics, education, health services, public health and social work.[39–42] Trials are a key source of the evidence used to inform evidence-based policy. Well-designed and conducted trials represent the most internally valid means of assessing the effects of complex interventions, by which we mean whether the results reported from a study are correct for the population within the trial.

So what are trials? Randomised controlled trials are experiments. They measure outcomes from people followed up after delivery of an intervention. They compare these outcomes between people who have been randomly allocated to receive the intervention versus those who have been randomly allocated not to receive it. The standard example of this is a trial of a new drug (e.g. to treat cancer) where half the patients enrolled in the trial are randomly chosen to receive the new drug and the other half receive a placebo. Differences between the two groups in, for example, death rates are then calculated.

But trials can be used to test interventions in the social world too. Imagine the example of a trial of whether providing women in poverty with access to small loans to set up a business helps them to keep their children attending schools. A trial might recruit a hundred women in poverty with school-age children. The women understand that they have a 50/50 chance of getting access to the loans and consent to participate. The women complete a baseline questionnaire asking questions about who they are, what they earn and own, how many children they have and whether these children are in school. Then, fifty women are randomly allocated to receive the loans and fifty are randomly allocated to act as controls. The intervention group gets access to the loans for whatever period of time the intervention involves. Those in the control group do not get this access but carry on with their lives as they would anyway. Then, after the intervention group has run for the required time, women in both groups are asked to complete follow-up questionnaires, asking similar questions as before. The trial analysis compares the rate of school attendance among the children of women in the intervention group with that among children of women in the control group. This example, like most 'standard' trials, involves random allocation of individuals. But trials can also randomly allocate 'clusters' of individuals: for example, schools. These are known as cluster randomised trials or, when geographic locations such as villages or communities are randomised, place randomised trials.

Randomisation tends to ensure (but does not guarantee) that the intervention and control groups are similar to each other at baseline. Crucially, this similarity applies not only to factors that are measured, for example, in a baseline questionnaire but also to unmeasured characteristics. Most importantly, randomisation prevents differences between the intervention and control groups in terms of how willing or able people are to engage with the intervention. If allocations were not random, certain kinds of people might select themselves into the new intervention group or the control group, and these differences would introduce what is known as 'selection bias'. The strength of trials reflects their capacity to allow a fair comparison between intervention and control groups. By 'fair comparison', we mean an estimate of the difference between an intervention group and a control group that is as attributable as possible to the difference in intervention receipt alone. Because the intervention and control groups in trials tend towards balance, the groups could be expected to experience comparable outcomes in the absence of intervention. In this sense, the control group makes for a 'counterfactual' of what might happen in the absence of intervention. Randomisation is a way to minimise bias. Ensuring a fair comparison reduces the chances that the results of the trial are actually the result of an unfair comparison.

Withholding an intervention from the control group might sound unethical but it is ethical if a number of conditions are met. Firstly, it is ethical if there is genuine uncertainty about whether the intervention is effective or not (known as 'equipoise').[43] For example, if we already know that loans for women in poverty do help the women keep their children in school, it would not be ethical to withhold these loans from the control group. But if this were the case, there might not be much point in evaluating the intervention at all. Secondly, it is ethical to have a control group the members of which do not receive the intervention as long as the members of this control group are still entitled to receive the normal range of interventions, services or support that are the normal standard of care. It is ethical to use trials to assess new interventions but it is not ethical to use trials to test established interventions because this would involve withdrawing entitlement to this normal standard of care from the control group. Thirdly, it is ethical if all those participating have consented to do so, based on their understanding what is involved (including that they may not get the intervention).

As well as random allocation, trials use several other methods to ensure that bias in the estimation of intervention effects is minimised. Firstly, trials use allocation concealment. This means that those who are allocating people or clusters to intervention versus control cannot 'game' the system. They cannot ensure that certain individuals or clusters do or do not receive the intervention. For example, if a doctor is randomly allocating patients to intervention or control, allocation concealment ensures that the doctor cannot subvert the system by opening the envelopes containing allocations so that they can give the intervention to patients who are more likely to adhere to the treatment.

Secondly, as in the example already described, trials generally collect baseline (pre-allocation) data as well as follow-up (post-intervention) data. Baseline data can be used to check whether there are major differences that have occurred by chance in the composition of intervention and control groups. If there are differences, these can be adjusted for statistically.

Thirdly, trials should as far as possible be 'masked' (or, as we used to say, 'blinded') so that those delivering interventions, those receiving interventions and/or those collecting and analysing data do not know whether a certain individual or cluster is in the intervention or control group. This is so that any such awareness does not bias the trial. Participants might report more positively on outcomes if they know they are in the intervention group. Intervention providers, data collectors or statisticians might consciously or unconsciously bias their work if they know who is in which group. Masking of providers and recipients is possible in most drug trials because those allocated to the control group can receive a placebo pill so neither the doctor nor the patient is aware of whether the patient is in the intervention or control group. This is why drug trials are sometimes described as being 'double masked' or 'double blinded'. However, in trials of other sorts of intervention (including most complex interventions), such masking is not possible. It would not be possible, for example, in a trial of a new school sex education intervention to mask teachers or students to whether they are receiving the new sex education intervention or are using the previous normal practice. But such trials can usually still mask data collectors and statisticians to allocation so that this does not bias their work.

Fourthly, trials should use validated measures so that they measure the thing they are intending to measure. If a trial is aiming, for example, to measure alcohol consumption, it should use a questionnaire or a diary method to collect this information for which there is evidence that the measure successfully captures how much alcohol someone is drinking.

Fifthly, how trials are done, analysed and reported should be guided by written protocols, drafted and made public before they begin. These protocols ensure that trials are conducted well and report transparently all their planned analyses. Without such protocols, it is possible, for example, for trial researchers to drop measures that do not indicate benefits or to cherry-pick outcomes that do suggest an effect.

Sixthly, the main analyses that are conducted on trial data should be what is known as 'intention to treat' rather than 'on treatment'. Intention to treat analyses include all allocated individuals or clusters in the analysis regardless of whether they actually fully received the intervention. In contrast, 'on treatment' (also sometimes known as per protocol) analyses only include those individuals or clusters allocated to the intervention who actually received this. While the latter might intuitively seem a fairer test of an intervention, it can actually bias results. This can happen when those allocated to the intervention group who do not receive the intervention are different to those who do receive it. Those who don't receive the intervention might be less healthy or less health conscious for example. If the analysis excludes such individuals from the intervention group but does not exclude any individuals from the comparison group, this will make for an unfair comparison. Intention to treat analyses introduce no such bias but may somewhat underestimate intervention effects if a substantial proportion of those allocated to an intervention do not actually receive it. For this reason, while the primary analyses which are done on a trial should be intention to treat,

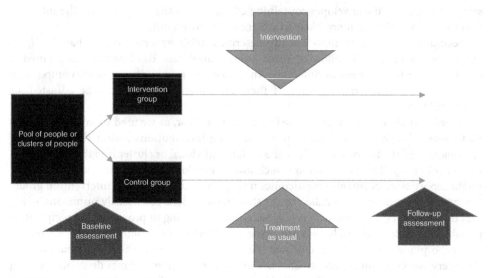

Figure 2.1 Randomised controlled trial

it may also be useful to conduct secondary on-treatment analyses. The randomised trial design is summarised above in Figure 2.1.

Because of all the aforementioned factors, randomised trials provide rigorous statistical estimates of the effects of allocation to an intervention versus a specific comparator condition on specific outcome measures among a specific population. In this sense, they offer a high degree of scientific rigour as a method. However, a single study is unlikely to provide a strong enough evidence base to inform health policy. The trial may have methodological limitations or it might involve quite a small sample. A single trial will also focus on a particular setting, population and point in time, which are unlikely to be representative of other places, people or time points. For this reason, researchers prefer to review the results of multiple studies, which brings us to consider systematic reviews.

2.2 How Do Systematic Reviews Work?

Systematic reviews have increasingly come to be recognised as the most comprehensive means of collating evidence from multiple evaluation studies. These reviews aim to summarise all of the evidence about a specific question: in this case, the effectiveness of a particular intervention versus a particular comparator for a particular outcome in a particular population.[44]

Previously, unsystematic reviews were conducted which aimed to summarise the overall evidence. However, these reviews were often criticised for not being transparent about what sorts of studies should be included, not being comprehensive in searching for all such studies, being selective so that they tended to include evidence that aligned with an author's prior views, not properly assessing or accounting for the size and quality of studies in summarising the evidence and not being transparent about how the results of studies were pooled and summarised to generate overall conclusions about effectiveness.[45]

In contrast, systematic reviews are transparent and clear about what questions they are trying to answer and hence what studies are pertinent to answering these questions, and pre-plan the methods for doing this in a way that reduces the risk of bias in reviewers' conclusions. They comprehensively use multiple methods to track down all the relevant studies. They systematically extract data on study sample size, methods and results and then assess study quality using validated tools. They use statistical and narrative methods to pool and summarise evidence on the effectiveness of interventions. Moreover, this process is carried out by a team of researchers so that discrepancies are identified and corrected. Systematic reviews commonly use what are known as 'meta-analysis' methods. These, in effect, pool the statistical evidence from across individual studies. This is a bit like creating a mega-trial with a much larger sample to estimate more precisely an intervention's effects. By pooling data from only the most pertinent and well-conducted trials, systematic reviews aim to offer not only more precise but also more comprehensive estimates of intervention effects. Because methods for doing systematic reviews are pre-planned, they minimise bias introduced by reviewers' selection of studies or 'cherry-picking' the literature. So, again in the sense of minimising bias, systematic reviews are our most scientifically rigorous method for summarising evidence. Despite the strengths of randomised trials and systematic reviews described in this section, there can be challenges in undertaking them, as well as limitations in the evidence they produce, which we now consider.

2.3 Challenges with Undertaking Randomised Trials

Trials may sometimes be difficult or even impossible to conduct. Those who provide or receive an intervention may reject the use of control groups because they see it as denying intervention to those who need it. They might believe in the effectiveness of the intervention even if it has not been subject to rigorous evaluation. Counterarguments from evaluators that it is ethical to withhold an intervention from a control group if we do not know whether it is effective, ineffective or harmful may not persuade anyone to change their mind. These issues might be particularly acute with interventions that are associated with strong personal beliefs, such as some forms of psychotherapy and community development.[46] [47] Sometimes equipoise genuinely is more complex. There might be clear evidence that an intervention is effective in terms of one outcome but not other important outcomes.

For example, in the run up to one study, the effects of childhood vaccine for individual risk of getting pneumonia were known but not its effects on the overall population rate of disease. This made it unethical to use a control group to evaluate these population impacts.[48] Similarly, if the impacts of an intervention on income or legal rights are known but not its health impacts, then again control groups may be unethical.[22] Sometimes an intervention is already being delivered as standard care. It would then be unethical to withdraw provision from a control group even if there is uncertainty about its impacts.[47] Control groups will also be impossible when it is necessary for legal, bureaucratic or practical reasons to deliver an intervention across an entire state or other area. This can mean that control groups are difficult to use in evaluation of mass media interventions, laws or welfare provision.[22]

There might be acceptance of using a control group but opposition to using random allocation to assemble the intervention and control groups. Practitioners might reject random allocation because they believe it prevents them from using their professional judgement to decide who should get the intervention. Policymakers might also reject random allocation because they have already decided or want to decide where/to whom an intervention will be delivered before the evaluation has started.[49] They may wish to see their new intervention implemented for the most promising or the most needy individuals or clusters first.[28] This latter scenario was the case in our evaluation of the youth work intervention delivered in England to prevent teenage pregnancy. The Department of Health insisted on using a competitive tendering exercise to decide which youth work agencies would pilot the intervention. This meant that we had to construct our control group comprising those agencies that did not win a tender. This is likely to have biased our evaluation towards identifying intervention benefits because the intervention group was likely to have higher baseline capacity to deliver good work than controls. It was therefore particularly surprising that our evaluation identified higher pregnancy rates in the intervention than control arm, and this increased our confidence that this was a real effect of a harmful intervention.[11]

Tracking participants from pre-intervention baseline measures to post-intervention follow-up outcomes can also sometimes be impossible, with or without a control group. This can be the case when, for whatever reason, an evaluation begins only after delivery of an intervention has started. Problems with tracking participants might also arise when policy-makers aren't willing to wait long for results. Tracking can be particularly difficult when there is a big gap between an intervention being delivered and outcomes then manifesting.[50] In short, trials are not always possible. When they are not possible, other designs can be used. In Chapter 6, we consider the strength of evidence that alternative designs can provide.

2.4 Limitations in the Evidence that Trials and Systematic Reviews Produce

Even where trials can and are conducted, there can be important problems and limitations in the evidence which they produce or in how this evidence is summarised within systematic reviews. One problem previously mentioned is that trials can sometimes neglect the evaluation of harm. This is particularly the case for 'harmful externalities' (because trials may not set out to measure these impacts) and in trials of public health interventions (because there is less appreciation of how these can cause harm).[17] When potential harms are not being assessed consistently across trials, systematic reviews cannot pool evidence on them.[17][51] This is an important gap because some harms, such as suicides, are rare enough not to be detectable in single trials but might be detectable in systematic reviews pooling multiple such trials.

We now want to consider another limitation of trials and systematic reviews as they are currently conducted, which will be a major focus for the rest of this book. Trials and systematic reviews have been heavily and rightly criticised for failing to open the 'black box' of how, for whom and under what circumstances interventions work. The criticism goes like this. Trials and reviews are a scientifically rigorous means of estimating, with as little bias as possible, the quantitative effects of a particular intervention on a particular outcome among a particular population. In other words, they successfully answer the input/ output question of 'Did intervention x raise the probability of outcome y among population z?'. However, trials and systematic reviews don't try hard enough to understand what comes in between the input of the intervention x and the output of outcome y. They don't examine the underlying processes of how the intervention is implemented or the underlying mechanisms by which it generates (or fails to generate) its outcomes. They do not consider how these processes and mechanisms vary for different people and places.

Exploring such differences in effectiveness might not be a problem if the intervention works the same for all. This might be the case for some biomedical interventions (though this should not be assumed[52]). It might even be the case for some complex interventions, such as parenting interventions to prevent childhood problem behaviour, which do seem to have quite similar effects across a variety of settings and populations.[53] However, it is unlikely to be the case for most complex interventions. Indeed, there has been a great deal of discussion in some disciplines, such as medicine and psychology, of a 'replication crisis', whereby the results of studies, including intervention studies, are not consistent when the studies are done in different places or with different populations.[54]

Remember our earlier definition of 'complex interventions', which focuses on their having multiple components which interact with each other and with the contexts in which they are delivered. In Chapter 1, we examined how the Intervention with Microfinance for AIDS and Gender Equity intervention to prevent HIV and gender violence included multiple interacting components and we explored how youth services interventions appear to have different effects on teenage pregnancy rates depending on where and to whom they are delivered. Most complex health interventions are likely to have different effects across different populations and settings. The first reason for this is that local factors will shape how well interventions are delivered. The second reason is that, in different areas, different sets of local factors will be causing the outcomes that the interventions aim to address.[55] For example, a US trial in the early 1990s reported on the effectiveness of an intervention training gay men to act as peer educators in their local communities to advise other men about the risks of HIV infection and how safer sex could reduce these risks.[56] However, UK trials of similar interventions from the late 1990s reported a lack of effectiveness.[57] These differences in results may have reflected more challenges implementing peer education in the UK settings.[58 59] But they may also have reflected differences in the local mechanisms influencing gay men's vulnerability to HIV. Lack of knowledge was a likely 'aetiological mechanism' influencing risk of HIV infection in the early 1990s, which could be 'disrupted' by peer education. In the later 1990s, other factors such as drug use may have been more critical aetiological mechanisms,[8] which were not likely to be 'disrupted' by peer education. Unless we understand why these differences in effect happen, it is very difficult for policymakers to decide when they should implement a certain intervention to address a certain outcome in a certain population and setting.

In particular, 'realist evaluators' and others have criticised conventional trials and systematic reviews for taking an oversimplified view of causality and not exploring how this emerges from the interaction of intervention mechanisms with the local context.[60 61] Effect sizes may tell us that an intervention helped more people than it harmed in a particular time and place. But without attending to how and for whom interventions work, they may not provide much help to policymakers and practitioners thinking through whether an intervention should be applied in other settings or for other populations.[62] Furthermore, focusing only on overall effects can also mean a neglect of the effects of interventions on health inequalities between different subgroups and how to reduce these.[63]

The conventional approach to conducting randomised trials can be criticised not only for not providing policymakers and practitioners with enough information but also for not being scientific enough in orientation. What we mean by this is that currently many trials are not orientated towards testing and refining our scientific theories about how outcomes are generated and how interventions might change this.[64] In effect, many current evaluations are really just a very rigorous form of descriptive monitoring. They describe intervention effects and might allow us to accredit some interventions as effective (at least in one time and place). This focus on accreditation is quite explicit in the work of clearing houses for effective interventions which generally offer little guidance about how, for whom and where interventions are likely to work.[65] Another way of putting this is that trials designed to estimate intervention effects have rightly focused on questions of 'internal validity' (whether the results reported from a study are correct for the population within the trial) but have neglected questions of 'external validity' (i.e. the implications of study findings for other settings and populations).[66]

As with trials, systematic reviews frequently synthesise only quantitative evidence of effect estimates in order to answer questions about 'what works'.[60 67] Methods such as meta-analysis are used to pool statistical measures of effect across the included studies to derive overall effect sizes. This assumes that there is a single overall effect across samples and that any variation largely reflects variation in the samples that studies recruit. This might be useful if an intervention really does work the same across populations and settings but not if such effects vary, as is likely to be the case with most complex interventions. Like trials, traditional systematic reviews do not 'open the black box' to assess how intervention mechanisms interact with context to generate outcomes. By presenting an overall effect across studies, they present a de-contextualised result which hides the variation caused by being implemented in different places or with different populations. This hinders not only assessments of transferability but also the development of future interventions.

This cursory summary of the shortcomings of trials and systematic reviews is a little unfair. Many trials increasingly do include embedded process evaluations aiming to describe how interventions are delivered. These process evaluations use a mixture of quantitative data (such as from client surveys, observation checklists and practitioner self-audits) and qualitative data (from interviews, focus groups and observations) to describe processes of intervention planning, delivery and receipt, as well as the contextual factors which affect this.[68] Occasionally, though rarer, process evaluations also use qualitative research to explore the mechanisms by which interventions might generate outcomes.[2] While these can offer important insights into how interventions work, they cannot make very definitive conclusions solely based on these data. For example, a process evaluation of a peer-delivered sex education intervention in England concluded from qualitative data that wider school context might influence the quality of peer education. The formality of school culture seemed to affect peer educators' own delivery styles.[69] But the qualitative results alone could not offer definitive evidence as to whether such factors affected the pattern of outcomes across schools.

Some trials do examine how effects vary between subgroups, defined in terms of characteristics of people or places, often to assess the impacts of interventions on health inequalities. Some even use what are called mediation analyses to see if an intervention achieves its impact on a certain health outcome via an intermediate effect on an intermediate outcome. For example, mediation analyses have tested if an intervention that reduces gender-based violence in schools achieves that effect by challenging violence-condoning norms.[70] Similarly, systematic reviews sometimes examine how intervention effects vary by the demographic profile of clients,[71] the use of specific intervention components,[72] or the context in which interventions are delivered.[73] These are all useful and are likely to provide important insights into how and for whom interventions work, and how well they might transfer to other populations and settings. However, our argument is that using some of these approaches without the others, or without an overall orientation to testing and refining our theories about how interventions work, will only provide limited insights into how interventions that work in one context have the potential to work in others.[55]

We have seen in this chapter that realist evaluators have been prominent in identifying the current limitations of trials and systematic reviews in generating useful evidence. In Chapter 3, we will explore what is meant by realist evaluation and realist synthesis, and consider what lessons we can take from this realist critique and alternative manifesto for evaluation and evidence-based policy.

Realist Critiques and Manifesto for Evaluation and Reviews

In this chapter, we examine an alternative approach to evaluation, known as realist evaluation, and assess what we can learn from this approach.

3.1 The Realist Approach to Evaluation

Realist evaluation was first developed by the criminologists Ray Pawson and Nick Tilley,[61] influenced by the critical realist philosophy of Roy Bhaskar.[74] [75] Pawson and Tilley argued that trials are misguided in focusing on *whether* interventions work, because, they argued, most interventions will work for some people under some conditions, and what evaluations really need to do is explore who these people are and what these conditions are. As an example of how uninformative trials can be, they cited the example of trials of mandatory police arrest for domestic violence, which aim to reduce rates of repeated assault.[76] The first trial of this in Minneapolis found a significantly lower rate of repeat calls for domestic violence among those random-ised to be arrested. But later trials reported mixed findings, with some even showing increased rates of repeat domestic violence among the intervention group. Pawson and Tilley suggested that these variations in effects could be understood by thinking about variations between the trial sites in the structure of local communities, employment rates and family structures. They suggested that arrest was a greater source of shame, and therefore a more powerful inhibitor of repeat offending in those contexts with stronger communities and more conventionally 'pro-social' norms.[61] In less stable or cohesive communities with less pro-social norms, arrest was not a powerful driver of shame or inhibitor of repeat offending.

Pawson and Tilley, and subsequently other realist evaluators, argue that instead of examining 'what works', evaluations should examine 'what works, for whom, under what conditions and how'.[61] They argue that interventions do not produce outcomes directly. Instead, interventions introduce new resources into, or redistribute existing resources within, a setting. These resources might, for example, involve money, materials, informa-tion or support. People in those settings (e.g. service providers, service clients or community members) might then use these resources to think or act differently.[77] The way they use these resources might then trigger mechanisms, and it is these mechanisms, not the intervention per se, which might then generate the intended outcomes, and/or perhaps some unintended 'outcomes'.

In doing so, these mechanisms might interact with other mechanisms that are present in the local context. For example, teachers might use curriculum resources to enact sex education lessons. Students might also participate in the enactment of these lessons. As a result, various

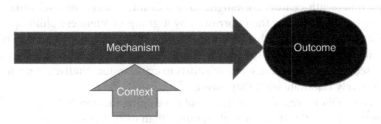

Figure 3.1 Context–mechanism–outcome configuration

mechanisms might be triggered which then generate outcomes. These mechanisms might involve students improving their knowledge about sexual health, changing their attitudes to particular aspects of sex (such as consent or contraception) or developing new skills (such as negotiating consent or successfully accessing or using contraception). In turn, these mechanisms might influence how the students decide when to have sex, and how they negotiate and enact sexual encounters. These mechanisms might interact with myriad other mechanisms operating within the local context, such as how local norms about gender and sexuality influence sexual encounters or how the local economy influences decisions about the timing of sexual debut or parenthood for different students. Realist evaluators propose that the focus of evaluation should be on understanding how the mechanisms triggered by deployment of intervention resources interact with features of the context to generate outcomes. These are understood in terms of context–mechanism–outcome configurations (CMOCs, Figure 3.1).

Informed by Roy Bhaskar's critical realist philosophy,[74][75] realist evaluators suggest that we need to understand the world in terms of various 'realms'. The 'empirical' realm consists of how we experience the world through our senses (and, in the case of researchers, our data). The realm of the 'actual' consists of events in the world, whether or not these are observed. The realm of the 'real' consists of the (unobservable) causal mechanisms which generate events in the world. These realms are often summarised as corresponding to experiences, events and causes, respectively.

Although not all realist evaluators are against the use of trials within realist evaluation,[78] many if not most are.[37][38][61][79] Some realist evaluators argue that it is misguided to try, as they believe trials do, to understand intervention effects merely in terms of observed 'constant conjunctions' of causes (allocation to an intervention) and effects (the outcomes) in the 'empirical' realm. They refer to this approach as being 'successionist'. Instead, they call for a 'generativist' approach which aims to understand what is going on in the realm of the 'real' in terms of how mechanisms generate outcomes. Causal mechanisms, they argue, involve 'tendencies' for causation but whether outcomes are generated depends on how these interact with other factors. Mechanisms might, for example, be triggered but cancelled out by other mechanisms or may not be triggered at all, depending on local circumstances. Because of this, realists argue that a lack of 'constant conjunction' does not necessarily disprove our theories about how mechanisms generate outcomes.[74][80] Therefore, instead of examining patterns of conjunction between allocation to an intervention and an outcome, evaluations should instead aim to build and refine hypotheses in the form of CMOCs.[61]

Some realist evaluators also criticise the use of trials on the grounds that these reflect a 'positivist' approach to understanding the world.[38][61] The term 'positivist' was originally coined by a nineteenth-century sociologist named Comte to describe a scientific approach to analysing society, and was then borrowed by a group of Viennese philosophers called 'logical positivists' who argued that only statements verifiable through logic and observation were meaningful.[81] [82] These days, the term is rarely used by anyone as a self-description but instead is used as a way for some social scientists to criticise quantitative research, although such critics rarely elaborate what they mean.[37] [61]

Pawson and Tilley stress the importance of developing theories in the form of CMOCs and then testing these. But they advise that, rather than using trials comparing an intervention group to a control group, tests should draw on 'observational' data: cases of interventions being delivered in real-life circumstances not controlled by evaluators. Pawson and Tilley argue that trials are bad science because real experiments in natural sciences, such as physics, do not employ control groups to explore the counterfactual (what would happen in the absence of intervention). Pawson and Tilley point to lab experiments to illustrate this. For example, in his experiments examining the motion of pendulums, Christiaan Huygens manipulated factors such as the length of the string and the point at which a pendulum is released to test his hypothesis about what factors influence the pendulum's motion.

Pawson and Tilley also criticise the use of control groups for aiming to strip away context in order to isolate an intervention's causal effects, bracketing out all other influences. They see this as running counter to the need to understand how mechanisms generate outcomes by interacting with context. A further concern expressed by some realists is that trials are so tightly controlled that they do not encompass sufficient diversity of contexts (e.g. in terms of people or settings) to allow for the proper examination of CMOCs.[37] This concern reflects a broader criticism that many trials and other research fail to recruit a diverse enough group of participants so that the studies cannot asses the effects of interventions on various subgroups, including marginalised or disadvantaged communities.[67]

3.2 An Example of a Realist Evaluation

We will reflect on these criticisms later in this chapter. For now, let us move on to consider an example of how realist evaluation might operate. Pawson and Tilley sketch out a hypothetical example of a realist evaluation of the impact of closed-circuit television (CCTV) in car parks as a way to prevent car theft.[61] To do this, realist evaluators would first develop some theories in the form of CMOCs about how this might work. One way that car theft could be prevented by CCTV would be by this enabling the 'arrest and removal' from circulation of car thieves. Another way would be for CCTV to encourage greater use of car parks and therefore create more 'natural surveillance', which would deter car thieves. Realists then insert a consideration of context into these theories. In some contexts, a few very active offenders might account for most thefts so the 'arrest and removal' mechanism might generate major impacts. This mechanism would likely be less important in contexts where a large number of occasional offenders operated. In car parks where usage, and therefore natural surveillance, is low, the 'natural surveillance' mechanism might be very impactful, but in contexts where usage is already high, this mechanism might be less important. To assess the validity of these CMOCs, Pawson and Tilley recommend a series of observational studies drawing on routine car theft statistics from a range of carparks in which CCTV has been installed, not at the behest of evaluators but as a matter of everyday policy by those managing these sites. It might be that these data indicate that the 'arrest and removal' CMOC was correct; the mechanism works in sites where police know that a core group of offenders are behind the thefts but not in sites where a larger group of occasional offenders are the problem. The evaluation might indicate that the 'natural surveillance' mechanism was not correct. There might be no evidence of a steeper decline in thefts in car parks that were little or much used at baseline. Later in this chapter, we reflect on these proposals for using observational data to test CMOCs.

3.3 The Realist Approach to Reviewing Evidence

Realists have criticised and offered an alternative not just for trials but also for systematic reviews. Systematic reviews, as with trials, are criticised for focusing on overall effects and trying to examine these using a successionist logic, pooling the effect sizes from multiple studies. Realists offer 'realist reviews' as an alternative. As with realist evaluations, realist reviews are orientated towards developing and testing CMOCs.[61] Realist reviews involve two stages. The first stage involves 'theory tracking': aiming to define CMOCs. The second stage involves 'theory testing': aiming to test and refine CMOCs. Systematic reviews define a research question and use this to define which narrow group of empirical studies are pertinent to answering this question, then conducting comprehensive searches for all such studies. In contrast, realist reviews draw on diverse sources, such as academic theory, descriptions of intervention theories of change and empirical research, to 'track' and 'test' the CMOCs.

Rather than aiming to include all empirical evidence fitting with defined inclusion criteria, the realist review instead aims to include a diversity of perspectives. The reviewers take particular findings here and there from included studies which shed light on tracking or testing the CMOCs. The research question is permitted to evolve as the included evidence sheds light on the nuances of the problem that the review is considering. Realist reviewers generally also do not use prescribed quality-assessment criteria because realists view quality assessment of an overall study as inappropriate given realist reviewers' interest in taking particular findings from a study. Realist reviews do aim to assess the quality of evidence but view this as requiring their expert judgements of particular findings rather than the use of standard checklists and assessing an overall study's rigour. Realists have developed a reporting standard for their reviews. This requires that reviewers explain and justify their judgements about the use of particular pieces of evidence.[83] The standards state:

> Within any document, there may be several pieces of data that serve different purposes, such as helping to build one theory, refining another theory and so on. Therefore, the selection (for inclusion or exclusion) and appraisal of the contribution of pieces of data within a document cannot be based on an overall assessment of study or document quality.   (p. 809)

When it comes to analysis, realist reviews aim to assess CMOCs in a quite different way to how traditional systematic reviews test hypotheses about effectiveness. Meta-analyses within systematic reviews test hypotheses by examining whether statistical differences between groups in study data are as would be predicted by hypotheses (e.g. the intervention is effective in terms of a certain outcome). In contrast, realist syntheses focus on *narratives*, assessing the plausibility of the narratives contained within CMOCs in light of the narratives offered by included study findings, refining CMOCs as necessary so that they account for these findings. Whereas conventional systematic reviews pool data from included studies using statistical meta-analysis (as well as writing narrative summaries of included studies), realist reviews instead aim for 'saturation'. This is achieved when the inclusion of more studies does not generate new insights, as the originators of realist reviews explain:[84]

> A decision has to be made not just about which studies are fit for purpose in identifying, testing out or refining the programme theories, but also about when to stop looking – when sufficient evidence has been assembled to satisfy the theoretical need or answer the question. This test of saturation, comparable to the notion of theoretical saturation in qualitative research, can only be applied iteratively, by asking after each stage or cycle of searching whether the literature retrieved adds anything new to our understanding of the intervention and whether further searching is likely to add new knowledge.   (p.28)

3.4 Are Realist Critiques and Alternative Approaches Correct?

We agree with much of the realist critique of trials and systematic reviews. And we agree with some of the suggested alternative approaches. We think the emphasis on developing and testing CMOCs is key. This should be useful in helping move evaluation from being a 'scientistic', pseudo-scientific form of descriptive monitoring to truly informing a science of complex interventions. However, we also think that some of realists' criticisms of trials and systematic reviews are wrong. And we think that the ways that realists aim to test and refine hypotheses within evaluations and reviews are often insufficiently rigorous. Here, we reflect on the aspects of the realist critique and the alternative with which we disagree, focusing largely on evaluation. In Chapter 7, we extend this consideration to realist critiques of, and alternatives to, systematic reviews.

Firstly, while we agree that statistical estimates of the overall effects of an intervention should not be the only information that evaluations provide, we think that they are often nonetheless useful. In the case of public health interventions in particular, scientists and policymakers are often very interested in whole-population impacts. The Rose hypothesis suggests that interventions delivered universally can often have larger overall population effects than interventions which target individuals at particular risk. Risk factors for non-communicable diseases are generally distributed with a bell-shaped curve (known as a 'normal' distribution) so that there are many more people at low or medium risk than high risk. This means that more cases of a non-communicable disease affect those deemed at low or medium risk rather than high risk (Figure 3.2).

Figure 3.2 shows how a universal intervention, by shifting the overall curve to the left, moves more people from higher into lower risk than does a targeted intervention: because more people are at medium or low risk than high risk. As a result, universal interventions can prevent more cases of a disease than can targeted interventions of similar effectiveness per individual.[85] For example, a trial of the ASSIST (A Stop Smoking in Schools Trial) peer-led smoking prevention intervention in UK secondary schools reported an overall effect of the intervention on smoking. The authors did this not because they believed that the intervention would have exactly the same effect on each student or in each school but because, in judging the success of public health interventions, they thought it would be useful to report the potential of the intervention to contribute towards population-level reductions in risk.[86] Even where the Rose hypothesis does not apply (either for public health interventions where risk is not normally distributed or for other sorts of interventions such as those addressing health care), it may still be a useful first step for an evaluation to determine overall effects before drilling down to examine what works for whom and where.

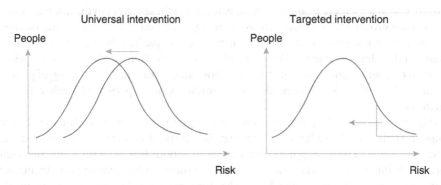

Figure 3.2 Rose hypothesis and how universal interventions can be more impactful

Secondly, we disagree that trials are, by definition and of necessity, too tightly controlled and insufficiently diverse to enable the proper testing of CMOCs. It is certainly true that some trials are insufficiently diverse.[52] But this is not a necessary or desirable feature, especially when assessing the effectiveness of complex health interventions, where the aim is often to ensure participants reflect the population from which they were recruited. When trials of such interventions aim to evaluate interventions in these kinds of 'real-world' conditions, they are often described as 'pragmatic' trials. In chapters 4, 5 and 6, we will describe our own trial of a school bullying prevention intervention and show both that this recruited a wide diversity of schools and students, and that this diversity enabled us to test a range of CMOCs. Furthermore, even if individual trials involve a relatively narrow range of settings and populations, we believe that systematic reviews can play a useful role in understanding why trial findings might be more positive in some contexts and less so in others. Indeed, we believe that, rather than indicating the limitations of trials, Pawson and Tilley's insightful interpretation of the various trials of mandatory police arrest for domestic violence actually indicates how useful trials can be and the potential for systematic review of these trials to shed light on how intervention mechanisms interact with context to generate outcomes.[61 76] Their interpretation that an intervention mechanism involving community shaming would only generate reductions in repeat offending in communities characterised by cohesion and pro-social norms was informed by their theoretically informed interpretation of findings from a number of trials.

Thirdly, we disagree with realists' rejection of the use of control groups. Pawson and Tilley's criticism that real science does not use control groups overlooks the fact that trials are used in many scientific areas, such as biomedical, environmental and agricultural sciences.[87] The realists' criticism fails to understand why control groups are needed for some experiments but not others. The use of a counterfactual is necessary within experiments when the experimenter cannot manipulate all of the factors involved. In Huygens' experiments on how pendulums work, the string length, the point of release and any other factor that will influence the pendulum's motion could be kept constant while others were allowed to vary. This is not the case in experiments involving complex health interventions. It would not be possible or desirable in a scientific study of the effects of sex education in schools to manipulate the profile of students in the school or the economic conditions of the towns in which the schools were located in the way it would in a 'laboratory' experiment. So instead, the experimenter accepts that there is going to be variation in these factors but tries to ensure that at least there is *similar level of variation* in these factors in the intervention and in the control group. Furthermore, it is worth recognising that sometimes evaluations hailed as exemplars by realists actually do involve control groups. This is the case with some of Pawson and Tilley's examples. One example is an evaluation of the effects of prisoner education on reoffending rates. The analysis draws on a control group made up of prisoners who moved through jail before the intervention, who experienced higher levels of reoffending.[61]

This brings us on to the purpose of the control group. We believe that the use of control groups in trials actually reflects not the stripping away of context as Pawson and Tilley contend but rather a proper appreciation that interventions interact with contextual factors in order to bring about an outcome. We believe that the outcomes among participants in the intervention group are generated by mechanisms triggered by the use of intervention resources interacting with myriad other mechanisms operating in that context. The outcomes among participants in the control group are generated by a similar array of contextual mechanisms but without the contribution of those specific mechanisms that would have been triggered by the use of the intervention resources. Thus, control groups allow the study to take proper account of the influence of context. They create the basis to 'bring them in' as opposed to 'bracket them out'. Crucially, the effect size does not represent impact in terms of reporting outcomes that were generated solely and uniquely by the intervention. Rather, it represents the *added value* of the mechanisms triggered as a result of the introduction and use of intervention resources to the sum of effects of all the mechanisms operating within the intervention group.

Fourthly, by rejecting consideration of counterfactuals, the model of realist evaluation proposed by Pawson and Tilley is extremely limited. It can only provide evidence of the plausibility of the effects of an intervention, not its precise probability.[88] To appreciate this, let us go back to the hypothetical example of the realist studies of CCTV impacts on car theft discussed in Section 3.2. We considered how studies might report that introduction of CCTV was followed by reductions in thefts in car parks, where the police knew that a small core group of offenders was behind the thefts but not in car parks with lots of thieves. These findings would thus suggest a plausible account of the arrest/removal mechanism being important but only in the context of a core group of offenders. Critically, however, in the absence of a randomised control group, these accounts don't tell us precisely how likely this conclusion is. It could be entirely wrong. For example, it might be that the downward trend in thefts in car parks where police knew that a core group of offenders was behind the crimes merely reflected 'regression to the mean' in these sites. In other words, the CCTV happened to be installed in these sites at a time of peak car crimes, which then drifted down to something nearer their normal level.

Similarly, we believe that realist syntheses fail to use sufficiently rigorous methods to examine causality. As we have seen, the testing of CMOCs within realist syntheses focuses on whether narratives described in included studies seem to align with the narratives encapsulated in the CMOCs being tested.[89] [90] For example, a realist review of how schools' tobacco policies influence student smoking included studies based on whether these provided a rich, detailed description of how policies might trigger mechanisms.[89] The review did not analyse whether the designs of some included studies meant that they offered more rigorous evidence of whether the introduction of smoking policies did lead to reduced smoking in certain contexts. The analysis reported in the review merely described each CMOC and then whether the narrative presented in each included study's conclusions supported this CMOC. No details were provided of these studies' methods or data. A broader analysis of realist reviews confirms this picture; few such reviews report how studies are appraised or how empirical findings are synthesised.[91]

Fifthly, we disagree with Pawson and Tilley's criticism of trials as inappropriately using a 'successionist' approach. The use of probabilistic statistics assessing associations between variables does not imply a belief that causation can only be inferred from constant conjunctions. Indeed, the use of statistics recognises that conjunctions are not constant. For example, an odds ratio reported from a trial represents the relative chance of a particular outcome among people allocated to an intervention compared to those allocated to the control group. If intervention and outcome were in constant conjunction, every single individual allocated to the intervention would experience the same outcome and every single person allocated to the control would not, so that the value of the odds ratio would be zero or infinity. Furthermore, statistical moderation analyses can examine how the association of two factors, such as study arm and outcomes, is contingent on the presence of one or more other factors. This enables, for example, an assessment of what works for whom. Statistical mediation analyses can assess whether the association between two factors (again such as study arm and outcomes) can be accounted for by a third intervening factor (such as an intermediate outcome), allowing for insights into whether an intervention works on a distal, or 'final', outcome, by changing outcomes on the way to the distal outcome. This can be used to explore the operation of mechanisms. While it is important to acknowledge that the realms of the empirical and the real are distinct, and therefore that mediators are not the same thing as mechanisms, such statistical analyses do nonetheless provide a useful means of examining whether our theories about mechanisms are valid.

Sixthly, we disagree with the broader criticism that trials (and quantitative research more generally) are necessarily positivist.[92] Those using this term, including realist evaluators, often do not fully explain what it means. Our reading of the philosophy of science and social science literature suggests that there are four tenets of positivism: (1) scientific knowledge derives from sensory observation; (2) theories must include concepts that align with empirical measures and not speculate about unobservable underlying mechanisms; (3) science aims to develop universally applicable laws; and (4) the natural and social sciences should use the same methods.[80] [93] We do not think that trials are of necessity positivist with regard to any of these four tenets.

With regard to the first tenet, trials generally operate within a 'hypothetico-deductive' approach to science rather than an inductive (theory-developing) or empiricist framework. In other words, trials do not hoover up data from the realm of the empirical in order to inductively build knowledge about the mechanisms operating in the realm of the real. Instead, evaluators plan a trial because they already theorise that the provision of certain intervention resources will enable the generation of certain outcomes. The theory is not directly built on data. Evaluators use their imaginations to develop the theories, informed ideally by prior academic theory and existing research.[39] Karl Popper, one of the key originators of the hypothetico-deductive approach, was very clear that this was an alternative to a 'naïve positivism', where experiments are the starting point for developing theories by induction:[25]

The fact that I have discussed the problem of social experiments before discussing ... the problem of sociological ... theories ... does not mean that I think observation and experiments are . . . logically prior to theories. On the contrary I believe that theories are prior to observations as well as experiments, in the sense that the latter are significant only in relation to theoretical problems. (p. 89–90)

With regard to the second tenet of positivism, we must admit that many trials are conducted either with very little prior theorisation of underlying mechanisms[94] or are informed by very superficial intervention theory, which is little more than a string of empirical measures connected by arrows denoting lines of causation.[94] However, this is not a universal or necessary feature of trials. Later in this book, we will describe our own trial of a school bullying prevention intervention. This used a theory of change that did go beyond empirical measures to theorise the deeper underlying mechanisms by which use of intervention resources in a school might ultimately lead to the generation of reductions in bullying. The theory was informed by deep sociological theory of the underlying mechanisms operating in schools.[95 96]

With regard to the third tenet of positivism, few trialists would explicitly claim that their results are universally generalisable: to do so would be not only positivist but also plain foolish. Guidance for undertaking health trials explicitly acknowledges that results from a trial may be an uncertain guide to wider effects.[97] When complex health interventions are transported from one setting or population to another, they are commonly subjected to a new trial in the new situation prior to wider use, implying a recognition that evidence of effectiveness in one context cannot be applied without scrutiny or reflection in other contexts. For example, the Family Nurse Partnership demonstrated benefits when trialled in the USA, but in England a trial reported it had no effect on smoking cessation, birthweight, rates of second pregnancies and emergency hospital visits for the child.[98 99]

However, we think that trialists' and systematic reviewers' actions (including, we must confess, our own sometimes) do imply an assumption that trial results are uncomplicatedly generalisable across contexts. As discussed in Chapter 2, most systematic reviews focus on quite general questions such as 'do health promoting schools interventions promote children and young people's health?'[100] Although these research questions specify a population (in this case, children and young people) and a setting (in this case, schools), they are very general. Furthermore, many meta-analyses fail to examine how intervention effects vary across what are often quite heterogeneous populations and settings.[53 100] This does seem to imply an assumption that the pattern of cause and effect is the same across studies, with any differences in effect sizes being largely the result of sampling and chance. However, these lapses in common sense do not demonstrate that an assumption of universal generalisability is a necessary or inevitable feature of trials or systematic reviews. For example, there are instances of trials and systematic reviews of violence and crime prevention interventions using subgroup analyses to provide more nuanced information about the contingency of intervention effects according to context.[73 101]

Concerning the fourth tenet, although trials clearly are used in both the natural and the social sciences, we think that trials of complex health interventions (which involve human interactions and actions) are very different from those used in fields such as environmental, agricultural and pharmacological sciences. The key distinction is that 'social science' trials should and increasingly do involve embedded qualitative research. This is significant because qualitative social science research is completely different in its goals to any research conducted in the natural sciences. Qualitative research focuses on humans as knowing subjects who interpret the world and engage in willed, socially meaningful actions quite unlike the objects of natural scientific research. Qualitative research is rooted in the 'hermeneutic' tradition, which aims to *interpret and understand* rather than *predict* human actions based on understanding how those involved give meaning to it.[102] Trials can draw on qualitative research for various purposes, most commonly to understand implementation. Informed by theory, such research can explore how providers and recipients of interventions make sense of these, commit to using them, work collaboratively with others to draw on intervention resources to act and then reflect critically on these processes to inform choices about subsequent actions.[103] [104] Furthermore, the quantitative measures that trials use are likely to better reflect participants' experiences and views if they are informed by prior qualitative research so that they engage with the world as it is socially constructed by people.[105] We believe the fact that randomised trials of complex social interventions include qualitative research – or use quantitative measures the development of which has been informed by qualitative research – therefore renders them completely different to randomised controlled trials used in the natural sciences. In Chapter 5, we will show how such qualitative analyses should be completely central to more scientific trials of complex health interventions.

We conclude that, while there are challenges with the current use of trials and systematic reviews of complex health interventions, and while some of the suggestions from realist evaluators are very useful, there are serious flaws in the realist critique of, and alternative to, trials and systematic reviews. We believe that the philosophy of critical realism and the use of realist evaluation approaches should not rule out use of trials or systematic reviews, and there may be more practical scope to examine CMOCs in trials and systematic reviews than many realists realise. We believe, in fact, that where trials and systematic reviews are feasible to conduct, they provide the most scientific rigorous means of examining questions of mechanisms and context while still enabling a rigorous assessment of causal attribution, which Pawson and Tilley's non-experimental approach lacks. In the following five chapters, we move on to consider how realist methods might be applied within trials and then systematic reviews to enable these to offer a more scientific approach to the evaluation of complex health interventions.

Chapter 4

Building Realist Theory in Evaluations

In this chapter, we start to describe how realist approaches might be used within trials of complex health interventions. We call this approach 'realist trials'. Some realist evaluators have criticised our approach, arguing that the term 'realist trials' is an oxymoron. They argue that trials are irretrievably positivist and successionist in their logic, and can never encompass sufficient diversity of sites and participants to allow testing of CMOCs. We hope that Chapter 3 sets out why we reject these arguments. Furthermore, we hope that, by describing in detail how realist trials should be used as a method, we will convince readers that this approach is feasible and useful. We start our consideration of realist trials by describing how these must first of all define a theory of change and develop CMOCs for the intervention being evaluated.

4.1 Theories of Change

First popularised by Carol Weiss, theories of change are intervention-specific theories about how intervention activities are supposed to generate intended outcomes.[2][106] Any intervention which involves undertaking some defined activities in order to achieve defined goals must have a theory of change even if, as was once common, this theory remains unstated. In the last few decades, intervention developers and/or evaluators have increasingly made their theories of change explicit. These are described either textually or using 'logic model' diagrams.[2] Logic models generally depict causal relationships flowing left to right from the deployment of intervention resources to intervention activities, intermediate outcomes and end outcomes, as in the hypothetical example shown in Figure 4.1.

Theories of change are useful in several ways. They enable intervention developers and providers to be clear about how they think an intervention will work. They make assumptions explicit and should allow potential weaknesses to be identified and fixed. There is some evidence that interventions with explicit theories of change are more effective than those lacking these.[107][108] Theories of change are also useful to evaluators in understanding what is the intervention that they are evaluating, and what measures they will need to assess to see if it has achieved its intermediate and/or ultimate outcomes.

Although interventions are increasingly informed by theories of change, these are very variable in sophistication and plausibility.[109] They often consist, like Figure 4.1, of various discrete constructs linked by arrows but with no consideration of either the underlying mechanisms that actually lie behind the arrows or how things might vary with context.[110]

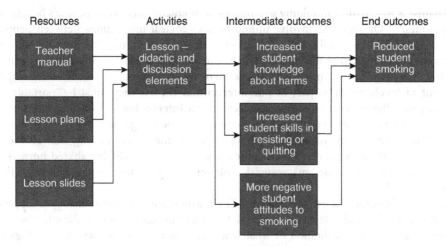

Figure 4.1 Example of a logic model for a school smoking prevention curriculum

Such theories are open to the charge, discussed in Chapter 3, that they are positivist because they restrict themselves to what are essentially a chain of quantitative empirical measures linked by arrows which do not really engage with mechanisms as they might be operating in the realm of the real. Logic models and theories of change can also fail to consider how mechanisms might play out differently in different contexts. There is no reference to context in Figure 4.1 for example. This can mean they do not fully consider how interventions work in practice or what benefits interventions aim to achieve for different groups and in terms of reducing health inequalities.

4.2 Theorising Mechanisms and Context

Realist evaluators have made a major contribution to improving theories of change, suggesting that these need to describe deeper mechanisms and that they need to propose how these mechanisms might interact with context to generate outcomes.[61][111] However, it should be recognised that other authors on evaluation have also similarly argued that theories of change should describe how intervention mechanisms interact with context to generate outcomes.[106][112–114] Including contextual factors within theories of change makes explicit our assumptions about how mechanisms might interact with context to generate outcomes. But it can also be useful in thinking through how an intervention needs to be designed to set off these mechanisms, by allowing optimal targeting and tailoring for different settings or populations, and ensuring implementation and organisational support for interventions. Being clear about how we think intervention mechanisms might interact with context to generate outcomes might help intervention developers and providers to ensure that an intervention is as effective as possible in as many contexts as possible.

Important questions to ask at this point are: what is a mechanism? and what is context? A large body of literature has considered the 'ontological' question of what do mechanisms consist of and how can we develop knowledge about them.[111] Informed by this literature, we see mechanisms as being distinct from, but triggered by, the way that providers or clients use intervention resources to enact an intervention. Providers and clients will change how they think and act, which may trigger other psychological or social changes.[61][103][111][115] Often, mechanisms will involve unfolding psychological interactions between people's beliefs and behaviours.[115] Or they will involve unfolding sociological interactions between people's agency (willed actions) and social structures (e.g. the local resources, institutions, communities or norms that can enable or constrain actions).[116] These mechanisms might operate at the individual, group, community, institutional or societal levels.[117] Because we develop an account of mechanisms as part of our intervention theory, they must be 'portable', or relevant to different groups of people receiving an intervention.[118] But mechanisms do not need to be relevant to everyone. Mechanisms can be categorised as involving macro-social influences on microsocial outcomes (e.g. the media influencing our attitudes); microsocial influences on microsocial outcomes (e.g. peers modifying shared norms); or microsocial influences on macrosocial outcomes (e.g. communities lobbying their politicians).[119]

So how can we know about mechanisms? This is a question about epistemology (as opposed to ontology). The realist literature suggests that mechanisms cannot be directly observed. Indeed, one influential definition of what is a mechanism describes these as 'ontologically distinct' from variables in this way.[118] Mechanisms exist in the realm of the real and are not the same thing as our evaluation data from the realm of the empirical.[61 75 120] However, evaluation data enable us to test our ideas about mechanisms and use these data to refine our theories. Some critical realist researchers have suggested that only qualitative research is nuanced enough to provide insights into mechanisms.[121] Other realist evaluators see a role for qualitative and quantitative research as shedding light on different aspects of how mechanisms operate.[61] We agree with the latter group, and, in the rest of this book, we discuss how this might occur within trials and systematic reviews.

And what is context? Context refers to the pre-existing set of organisational, community and other social structures; material, economic and informational resources; and norms and values within which an intervention is implemented. These might be attributes of individuals, or social groups or structures. Contexts contain myriad other biological, psychological and social mechanisms which themselves contribute to generating beneficial or adverse outcomes within a setting, and which interact with the mechanisms triggered by an outcome to generate its outcomes.[111] Contexts might affect how intervention mechanisms do or do not generate outcomes in different ways. This can include the extent to which people in the contexts have needs (i.e. 'vulnerabilities') that intervention mechanisms might address, such as a peer education intervention addressing lack of knowledge of HIV transmission. It can also include the extent to which contexts offer opportunities (i.e. 'affordances') either for the intervention being delivered or for supporting the mechanisms which the intervention is aiming to trigger, such as whether women receiving microfinance can use this to start a small business.[114]

Given contexts contain mechanisms and given contexts can obviously be reshaped as a result of intervention mechanisms,[122] some authors have suggested that there is a confusion within realist evaluation about the distinctions between contexts and mechanisms.[111 123] Our view, however, is that although mechanisms and context are not ontologically distinct phenomena (they are made of the same stuff), it is nonetheless useful to frame them differently when we define our CMOC hypotheses. Another way to think of this is that a given phenomenon (e.g. feeling safe) may be a feature of a certain context and it may be a mechanism in another. Context–mechanism–outcome configurations are merely tools for spelling out what we are hypothesising; they are not defining fixed, immutable categories of reality. In our teaching, we distinguish between context as that which people, communities and organisations bring to the intervention, and mechanism as that which happens when you bring interventions to people, communities and organisations on the way to generating an outcome. We use the terms 'context' and 'mechanism' so that we can frame propositions about how we think interventions work and use this to collect data to examine these propositions. Some evaluators influenced by critical realism have switched from using CMOCs to using configurations which also include agency, or to focusing instead on how interventions and contexts interact to trigger mechanisms which generate outcomes.[111] [124] We prefer to stick with CMOCs because we think these provide analytic clarity about how mechanisms operate. We do, however, recognise the importance of agency in both contexts and mechanisms.

4.3 The Case Study: A Randomised Trial of the Learning Together Intervention

In this and the next two chapters, we use our own evaluation of a school bullying prevention intervention as a case study to show how we go about conducting realist thinking and analyses within a trial. The intervention was called 'Learning Together' and was a 'whole-school' intervention, which means that it didn't just involve classroom teaching but also involved various activities across the whole school at different institutional levels. Learning Together provided secondary schools in England with various resources: a manual to guide intervention delivery in schools; a needs assessment report profiling each school's students in terms of their attitudes to school, experience of bullying and broader health based on data from annual student surveys; curriculum materials and lesson plans to deliver classroom teaching about social and emotional skills; training for teachers in using a technique called 'restorative practice'; and an external facilitator to support schools in coordinating the use of these resources in the first two years before school staff facilitated the intervention without external support in the third year.

The aim was that school staff and students could then draw on these resources to enact various activities. The first of these involved regular meetings of an 'action group' comprising staff and students supported by the manual and external facilitator. This group aimed to review the information on student needs and decided how to make the school a more engaging, inclusive and supportive place. Members were also tasked with revising school rules, policies and systems to support this. The second activity was staff using 'restorative practice' to address bullying and other conflicts. Restorative practice is a disciplinary method that does not merely punish offenders but also aims to enable victims to describe harms, offenders to take responsibility and both to build better relationships. The third activity was teachers delivering lessons on social and emotional skills in classrooms.

We will discuss the design of the evaluation of Learning Together in detail in later chapters. But, in short, the intervention was first evaluated in a small pilot study which randomised four schools to receive the intervention and two to act as controls for one school year. This study focused not on assessing outcomes but rather on assessing the feasibility and acceptability of both the intervention and the evaluation methods. The intervention was then refined and then evaluated using an explicitly realist cluster randomised controlled trial. Baseline surveys were completed with students at the end of year seven (which is the first year of secondary school when students are aged eleven to twelve years). Twenty schools were then randomly allocated to receive Learning Together and twenty to continue with their usual practice. Student surveys were repeated two and then three years later. During the three years when the intervention was enacted, a process evaluation used qualitative and quantitative methods to examine provision in intervention schools in terms of both implementation and mechanisms.[125] Control schools were also involved in the process evaluation. Using similar methods, we sought to understand their context and document what activities they were undertaking to reduce bullying and aggression. When we report any data from the Learning Together trials, all the names of schools or individuals are changed to ensure the anonymity of our participants.

4.4 Defining a Theory of Change

The first stage of our evaluation consisted of describing a theory of change for the intervention and using this to define some starting CMOCs.[126] Intervention theories of change should, where possible, be informed by middle range theory.[26] This is scientific theory about the general mechanisms (i.e. not necessarily concerning an intervention) that generate outcomes. This should be analytically general enough to apply to a range of settings, populations and/or outcomes, but specific enough to be useful in a given application. Such theory might specify contextual factors upon which these mechanisms are contingent.[25] Basing intervention theories of change on middle range theory should help us think through our assumptions about what resources we should provide and why. And if the middle range theory is itself supported by empirical evidence, this should also be a means by which interventions might be informed by broader scientific knowledge.[127]

But how do we choose an appropriate middle range theory on which to base an intervention's theory of change? Firstly, the middle range theory should not merely be retrofitted onto an existing intervention since this offers no possibility that the middle range theory can beneficially influence the intervention's design.[128] The middle range theory should have some empirical evidence, which suggests that it has validity, ideally from populations and settings and with regard to outcomes similar to those with which the intervention will engage. The middle range theory should describe mechanisms that could plausibly be triggered by the intervention in question. There is no point in using a middle range theory if the intervention couldn't plausibly trigger the mechanisms that the middle range theory suggests. If this is the case, either a different theory is needed or else the intervention must be adapted so that it could trigger the theorised mechanisms. And lastly, the theorised mechanisms should align with the needs or vulnerabilities of the target population if it is to generate benefits for them. In Chapter 3, for example, we considered HIV prevention interventions for gay men. We explored how a peer education mechanism might align with men's needs in a context when lack of knowledge is a critical factor affecting vulnerability to HIV infection but not when the context has been transformed and other factors are more important.[8]

Learning Together was informed by a middle range theory called the 'theory of human functioning and school organisation',[95] which was in turn informed by several other academic theories and pieces of scholarship.[96] [129] The theory of human functioning and school organisation proposes that it is possible to reduce student involvement in health-related risk behaviours (including bullying) by promoting student commitment to the school. This involves students increasing their commitment to the school's 'instructional order' (i.e. teaching and learning) and to the school's 'regulatory order' (i.e. discipline and community). In turn, this firstly requires that schools 'reframe' their provision so that this focuses on student needs. Secondly, schools need to 're-classify' school processes so that these erode various 'boundaries' within the school. This is a fancy way of saying that schools need to improve linkages between staff and students, between students' academic and broader personal development and between the culture of the school and its local community. The theory suggests that these mechanisms will be particularly beneficial for more disadvantaged students, for whom commitment to school is often not the default in the way that it might be for more privileged students. In other words, some students are likely to benefit from an intervention because they have needs or vulnerabilities which the intervention mechanisms can address.[8] This theory thus proposes a mechanism not only for benefiting individuals but also for addressing inequalities across individuals.

This theory seemed a good choice firstly because there was some empirical evidence that it was correct. Several studies had reported that students in schools that better engage students in learning and attendance were also less likely to report a range of risk behaviours, including violence.[130][131] It also seemed a good fit because it seemed plausible that involving students in action groups and restorative practice could erode boundaries between staff and students. Teaching students social and emotional skills might also erode boundaries between academic and broader personal development. These processes might therefore increase student commitment to school and therefore decrease health risk behaviours. And finally, there was some evidence that the mechanism set out in theory fitted with what students in England need; there was evidence that students' commitment to schools was not optimal but was likely to be protective if it were increased.[132]

So we drew on this middle range theory to develop our theory of change as depicted in Figure 4.2.

As well as being informed by existing academic theory, Learning Together and its theory of change were also informed by existing empirical research. For example, there was evidence that student participation in action groups could transform the commitment to school not just of the students directly involved but also of other students. These others students could come to feel more positively about school as a result of seeing it take steps to involve students in decision-making to make the school a more inclusive place.[133][134]

It can also sometimes be useful to undertake new 'formative' research specifically to inform an intervention and its theory of change. Such research can explore the local context within which an intervention is planned and existing mechanisms that appear to be generating outcomes in that context. Such formative research can employ purposive sampling to provide contextual diversity. An example of such research is a formative study used to inform the development of an intervention to promote safe sex and relationships among older adolescents in further education colleges.[135] Focus groups and interviews with staff and students were used to explore student and staff views on how an intervention might work to help students manage relationships and sexual health. Informed by this work, staff and students then completed questionnaires about how intervention mechanisms might interact with context to play out differently with different student groups or in different colleges.

It is also important for interventions and their theories of change to be informed by consultation and engagement with the public, practitioners and policymakers. In the health sector, such a consultation is often called 'patient and public involvement and engagement'. Citizens, practitioners and policymakers are likely to have insights into how intervention mechanisms might generate outcomes, and how these might play out differently in different settings or for different groups. We consulted with school staff, education policymakers and young people in the course of developing our plans for our original pilot study of Learning

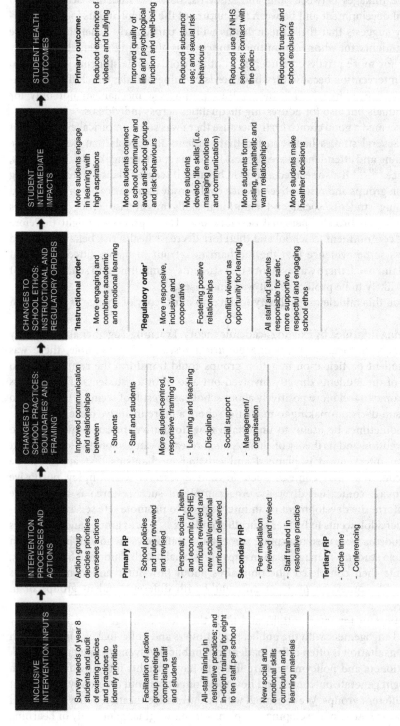

Figure 4.2 Logic model for Learning Together intervention

INCLUSIVE INTERVENTION INPUTS	INTERVENTION PROCESSES AND ACTIONS	CHANGES TO SCHOOL PRACTICES: 'BOUNDARIES' AND 'FRAMING'	CHANGES TO SCHOOL ETHOS: INSTRUCTIONAL AND REGULATORY ORDERS	STUDENT INTERMEDIATE IMPACTS	STUDENT HEALTH OUTCOMES
Survey needs of year 8 students and audit of existing policies and practices to identify priorities	Action group decides priorities, oversees actions	Improved communication and relationships between	**'Instructional order'**	More students engage in learning with high aspirations	**Primary outcome:** Reduced experience of violence and bullying
	Primary RP	- Students	- More engaging and combines academic and emotional learning		
Facilitation of action group meetings comprising staff and students	- School policies and rules reviewed and revised	- Staff and students		More students connect to school community and avoid anti-school groups and risk behaviours	Improved quality of life and psychological function and well-being
		More student-centred, responsive 'framing' of	**'Regulatory order'**		
All-staff training in restorative practices; and in-depth training for eight to ten staff per school	- Personal, social, health and economic (PSHE) curricula reviewed and new social/emotional curriculum delivered	- Learning and teaching	- More responsive, inclusive and cooperative	More students develop 'life skills' (i.e. managing emotions and communication)	Reduced substance use; and sexual risk behaviours
		- Discipline	- Fostering positive relationships		
	Secondary RP	- Social support	- Conflict viewed as opportunity for learning	More students form trusting, empathetic and warm relationships	Reduced use of NHS services; contact with the police
New social and emotional skills curriculum and learning materials	- Peer mediation reviewed and revised	- Management/ organisation	All staff and students responsible for safer, more supportive, respectful and engaging school ethos		
	- Staff trained in restorative practice			More students make healthier decisions	Reduced truancy and school exclusions
	Tertiary RP				
	- 'Circle time'				
	- Conferencing				

Together. Participants told us that restorative practice was of considerable interest to schools and education policymakers, with staff and students seeing this as having the potential to transform relationships between staff and students.

What should now be clear is that our theory of change was much more nuanced than what was described in the logic model shown in Section 4.1. Our logic model, like others, does not engage with how mechanisms are theorised to interact with context to generate outcomes. However, this omission is, in our case, merely to avoid making the logic model too visually complicated. To complement our logic model, we developed a textual theory of change informed by plausible and useful sociological middle range theory to describe the complex mechanisms that we hoped would generate reductions in bullying. It suggests that the intervention would generate reductions in bullying prevention by bringing about changes to how schools are organised, modifying school 'classification' and 'framing' in the way theorised by the theory of human functioning and school organisation. In turn, these would increase students' commitment to school, which would lead to reduced student involvement in anti-school peer groups and risk behaviours, including bullying.

4.5 Introducing Context: Defining Context–Mechanism–Outcome Configurations

The description in Section 4.4 of the theory of change and the middle range theory also hints at how mechanisms might interact with context. We have said, for example, that we expected the mechanisms to be more powerful in building student commitment to school among more disadvantaged students. We needed to spell this out explicitly and think through other ways in which context might play a role. To do this, we developed some starting CMOCs to supplement the logic model.

As well as using the theory of human functioning and school organisation to hypothesise that the intervention mechanisms were more likely to generate beneficial outcomes for socio-economically disadvantaged students, we also drew on empirical evidence to develop other CMOCs. For example, we hypothesised that implementation would have better fidelity and therefore be more likely to trigger our mechanisms when the school had the organisational capacity to implement it properly, for example, as measured by the school having a good recent rating by the national school inspectorate. This was informed by a previous realist review of what factors influence the implementation of school-based health interventions.[136] We also hypothesised that our theorised mechanisms were more likely to generate student benefits in schools in which the culture was already relatively inclusive (valuing and respecting all students). We hypothesised that, in schools with more authoritarian cultures (which aimed to control and coerce students into compliance with school rules), the mechanisms triggered by the intervention were likely to be swamped by other mechanisms. Another way of putting this is that some school contexts offered more opportunities or 'affordances' for intervention mechanisms.[114] Some school contexts were more likely to offer affordance for a mechanism increasing student sense of belonging because they had a pre-existing culture of offering students the chance of inclusion. Informed by existing qualitative research, we theorised that these other mechanisms would involve less educationally committed students further disengaging from authoritarian school cultures and instead committing to anti-school peer groups and risk behaviours as an alternative marker of identity, status and the transition to adulthood.[137]

4.6 Theorising Harms via 'Dark Logic Models'

As well as considering mechanisms by which beneficial outcomes are generated, we believe that theories of change and CMOCs should also consider potential harmful unintended outcomes. We have developed the concept of 'dark logic models' to develop hypotheses about such harms. We think this is important because, as we saw in Chapter 1, complex social interventions can generate unexpected harms via unanticipated mechanisms. These harms might be paradoxical effects (where the intervention causes harms in the very outcomes it is trying to beneficially impact) or harmful externalities (harms to altogether separate outcomes). Evaluations need to be guided by hypotheses about harm in order that we have in place measures for potential harmful externalities. Like theories of change intended to theorise how interventions might generate benefits, developing dark logic models for potential intervention harms should help intervention developers or providers to modify an intervention to reduce the risk of these harms being generated. Developing dark logic models should also help evaluators to be able to collect data on whether these harms do manifest and if so how and for whom.

A better understanding of how intervention mechanisms might generate harms should help ensure future interventions avoid such harms. For example, existing research suggests that some group interventions for young people, which aim to reduce risk behaviours such as drug use, can actually increase these behaviours. This can occur via interventions not being well facilitated so that interactions between participants provide positive peer reinforcements for pro-risk attitudes and behaviours.[12] This evidence should be useful in ensuring other interventions avoid such mechanisms. Establishing that a particular intervention can cause harm doesn't necessarily mean that the whole intervention needs to be abandoned. Understanding the mechanisms underlying harms can enable refinements of the sort Karl Popper envisaged with his idea of 'piecemeal social engineering' as discussed in Chapter 1.[138] To develop a dark logic model, evaluators should start with their logic model of how the intervention is meant to work so that its assumptions can be scrutinised and the 'dark logic' of potential harms be considered. We recommend using three approaches to build a comprehensive dark logic model.

Firstly, the potential mechanisms of intervention harm can be theorised by reflecting on possible interactions that might occur between, on the one hand, the 'agency' (freely willed actions) of providers or recipients and, on the other, the social structures that enable or constrain this agency. These structures might concern the policies or norms of the institutions or communities through which the intervention is delivered, the manuals instructing how the intervention should be delivered or the economic or other resources underpinning delivery. Reflecting in this way on how agency and structure might interact in unintended ways might also be informed by existing middle range theories. Applying this to Learning Together, we hypothesised that the emphasis in the intervention's manual on local decisions might interact with staff agency so that the interventions were 'hijacked' in some very academic schools to focus not on improving student health but rather on improving student academic attainment. This focus might then lead to lower school commitment and worse mental health among the least committed, less academically motivated students within these schools.

Secondly, potential mechanisms of harm might be theorised by evaluators comparing their intervention and its logic model to existing evaluations of similar interventions (or interventions aiming to trigger similar mechanisms). The intervention being developed might be compared to some interventions previously found to be effective and some previously evaluated as harmful to explore points of similarity and difference. This will of course only be possible if there is an extensive enough body of existing evaluation evidence to allow this. The comparison we have in mind is purely qualitative, with a view to refining the intervention and informing further hypotheses to assess whether there was evidence of harm. Applying this to Learning Together, we compared the restorative practice element of the intervention to other evaluations of restorative practice, which suggested that it is effective in addressing conflict.[139] But we also compared it to the broader literature on interventions which target young people based on their involvement in risk behaviours. Some of these report harms which probably arise via a mechanism of labelling participants as 'deviant' leading to the amplification of risk behaviours.[12] So we hypothesised that there might be a possibility that restorative practice leads some students to become more, not less, involved in bullying perpetration. After we had developed our CMOCs, we also became aware of a literature about potential harms in violence prevention interventions focused on the 'healthy context paradox'.[140] This suggests that school-based interventions that are otherwise successful at improving mental health by reducing violence might nonetheless worsen mental health for those 'leftover' pupils still experiencing bullying. We used the CMOCs implied by this theory as the basis for a later test of harms (see Chapter 8).

Thirdly, possible mechanisms of harm might be theorised by consultation and engagement with providers, policymakers and community members. These people will likely have insights into the settings in which the intervention will be implemented and how interventions might operate within these. Applying this to Learning Together, we found from some consultations that some school leaders were worried that the intervention's multiple components might make it too complex to implement in some schools, particularly those with low organisational capacity or confronting other challenges. We hypothesised that the intervention might disrupt existing provisions within schools with low capacity or experiencing other challenges, leading to increased student bullying.

4.7 Summarising Our Context–Mechanism–Outcome Configurations

In Box 4.1, we summarise the CMOCs that emerged from the thought processes in Sections 4.4, 4.5 and 4.6 prior to the study commencing.

Box 4.1 Summary of prior Learning Together CMOCs informed by the theory of change and other sources

Mechanism of Benefit

Context: Particularly among socio-economically disadvantaged students, and in schools with strong organisational capacities and inclusive cultures.

Mechanism: Learning Together resources enable reclassification and reframing in schools so that boundaries between staff and students, students' academic and personal development and the school and local community are eroded.

Outcome: Generating increased student commitment to school, reduced commitment to anti-school peer groups and decreased risk behaviours, including bullying.

'Hijacking' Mechanism of Harm

Context: Particularly among the least-committed students in the most academically oriented schools.

Mechanism: The emphasis in the intervention's manual on local decision-making enables the intervention to be 'hijacked' to focus less on improving student health and more on improving student academic attainment.

Outcome: Generating lower school commitment and worse mental health among some students.

'Labelling' Mechanism of Harm

Context: Particularly among repeat participants in restorative practice.

Mechanism: Participants come to perceive that they are being labelled as 'deviant'.

Outcome: Generating an amplification of risk behaviours, including increased bullying perpetration.

'Disruption' Mechanism of Harm

Context: Particularly among schools with low organisational capacities or experiencing other challenges.

Mechanism: Learning Together disrupts existing provision which has hitherto kept bullying from escalating.

Outcome: Generating worse not better bullying prevention leading to increased student bullying.

This chapter has described the importance of constructing theories of change for interventions which consider the mechanisms that the use of intervention resources trigger and how these mechanisms then interact with context to generate impacts both beneficial and harmful. Chapter 5 describes how these theories might be refined by drawing on empirical evaluations of the processes by which interventions are delivered and received.

Refining Realist Theory through Process Evaluations

In the previous chapter, we described how to define intervention theories of change and CMOCs before a trial starts. In this chapter, we consider how to refine them in the course of doing a trial, drawing on data from process evaluation. As the name suggests, process evaluations examine processes, not outcomes. They look at processes of intervention planning, delivery and/or receipt. Increasingly, they also look at the mechanisms by which interventions generate outcomes.[2] In phased approaches to evaluation typical in the United Kingdom, two separate process evaluations are generally conducted. The first occurs within an initial feasibility, or pilot study, which concentrates on questions of feasibility and acceptability. Feasibility and pilot studies are done before attempting to do a trial of effectiveness. Feasibility studies explore several specific areas of uncertainty, while pilot studies involve a dress rehearsal on a small scale for the later evaluation of effectiveness. Such studies are done because effectiveness trials are expensive, so we need to check that our planned interventions and evaluation are possible and refine our methods where necessary before we commit to evaluating effectiveness. The second time we run a process evaluation is as an integral part of an effectiveness trial. In this chapter, we first consider the general way in which process evaluations and, in particular, qualitative research done within process evaluations can be used to refine CMOCs. At the end of the chapter, we then consider the different roles of process evaluation in feasibility and pilot studies versus effectiveness studies.

5.1 Why We Need to Refine Context–Mechanism–Outcome Configurations

Using qualitative research to refine our theories of change and CMOCs is really important. It ensures that the hypotheses that we eventually test using quantitative trial data are as plausible as possible. Our initial theories, even if they are informed by the best middle range theory, empirical research and consultation, may still be sharply at odds with how things seem to be working in practice. So, qualitative research is useful as a reality check on our theory of change and CMOCs before we use them to derive hypotheses which we test statistically.

We do not want to test a very long list of hypotheses, and the ones we do want to test need to be good. So why do we want to test a reasonably parsimonious set of hypotheses? Our tests of hypotheses using quantitative data report a statistical probability of whether a certain pattern in the data (e.g. that allocation to an intervention is associated with an outcome) might have arisen by chance. A rule of thumb is that if these statistical tests of significance tell us that the chances of an association arising by chance are only one in twenty, then we might feel fairly confident that an association is statistically significant. The problem is that if we have tested twenty hypotheses in this way, then there is a good chance that at least one of the associations identified as significant will have arisen by chance.

So, we want to winnow down and hone our hypotheses before we test them. We want to throw out any hypotheses that just don't seem plausible in the light of our qualitative research. And we want to refine the remaining hypotheses so that we concentrate our limited statistical firepower on hypotheses we think are really plausible. Qualitative research is really useful in helping refine our theories of change and CMOCs. This is because qualitative research is open-ended, so it can raise possibilities that we previously hadn't considered.[141] Process evaluations collect qualitative data via individual or group interviews (the latter often called focus group discussions). These might involve intervention providers, recipients or other participants (such as policymakers, recipients' family members or others with some involvement with the intervention). It rightly treats such people as experts on the local context, how the intervention is being implemented and how it might be working.

Qualitative research conducted within process evaluations can be used post hoc to explain quantitative findings on outcomes. However, there is a risk that when using qualitative research to account for quantitative findings, such analyses are prone to confirmation bias whereby qualitative data are scrutinised for reasons for a particular quantitative finding, ignoring qualitative data which do not align with these quantitative findings.[68] We therefore think it is far better for qualitative research to occur first, building theory about mechanisms which can then be tested in subsequent quantitative analyses.

5.2 Qualitative Research within Process Evaluations

Qualitative research is completely different to quantitative research. We first referred to qualitative research in Chapter 3, where we described qualitative research as being rooted in the 'hermeneutic' tradition, which aims to *interpret and understand* rather than *predict* human actions based on understanding how those involved give meaning to it.[102] It doesn't ask people to complete tick boxes in multiple-choice questions with a (necessarily) restricted range of options. Instead, it involves an interviewer asking a series of questions, most of them open-ended, and all of them allowing the interviewee or the focus group participant to answer as they see fit.[93] This format allows for the possibility of finding out things we hadn't thought of when we planned the study. Qualitative research involves smaller samples than is commonly the case with quantitative research. It uses sampling aiming to generate a diverse set of experiences and views rather than a statistically representative group. This use of small samples is partly because the collection and analysis of qualitative data are more labour-intensive and costly, so we can't involve so many participants as quantitative research.

But, more importantly, it is because the purpose of analysis is not to assess the prevalence of a particular view or experience, or identify associations between different views and experiences. Instead, qualitative research aims to provide an interpretation of how different people describe their views and experiences.[93][116] It generally looks for themes within or across the transcripts of interviews with different people. These themes might involve different people, all describing similar experiences or views but using different languages. Or it might involve seeing a pattern whereby interviews themselves describe links between different views or experiences as a way for them to explain the world as they see it. Sometimes, we find apparent contradictions, where some participants see the world in one way, while others see it quite differently. The aim of the analysis is to develop an interpretation of the data which makes sense of it all. Some qualitative analyses aim to develop theory,[142] while others are content to provide a more descriptive analysis of themes.[93] Qualitative research generally aims to involve a sample diverse enough that the analysis achieves 'saturation': the point at which the analysis of more data doesn't move the analysis any further forward.

Process evaluation generally uses a mix of quantitative and qualitative research to examine questions of implementation, context and mechanisms.[2] It was originally developed largely as a quantitative check that interventions had been delivered as planned. This could help interpretation of the results of an outcome evaluation. For example, evaluators could check whether a lack of effect of an intervention on an outcome was due to the genuine incorrectness of the intervention theory of change (as applied to a particular context) or instead merely to a failure of implementation.[143] Over time, process evaluations came to broaden both their focus and methods. As well as fidelity, they examined questions of feasibility, reach and context. As well as quantitative data, they collected qualitative data from interviews, focus group discussions and researcher observations.[68] Process evaluations' ability to describe interventions has been aided by moves to encourage more standardised descriptions of intervention methods and processes.[144][145] Process evaluations have also become increasingly informed by theories of implementation. For example, Carl May's general theory of implementation guides process evaluators to examine how intervention providers and recipients understand an intervention, decide whether they want to commit to its delivery, work collaboratively with others to make it happen and then reflect on how it has gone and perhaps how things need to change to make it better.[103][104] Most recently, process evaluations have started to examine the mechanisms which generate impacts as well as processes of implementation.[2]

However, while the arguments for using qualitative research to examine and refine mechanisms are widely recognised, there is little detailed guidance on how to do this. The Medical Research Council frameworks for the evaluation of complex interventions and for process evaluation suggest some general principles about using process evaluation to examine mechanisms.[1][2] The process evaluation guidance, for example, suggests using qualitative research to explore mechanisms that are unanticipated and/or too complex to be captured quantitatively. However, the frameworks do not offer detailed guidance on how qualitative data might be sampled, collected or analysed in order to do this. We attempt to offer this in this chapter.

5.3 Different Approaches to Exploring Intervention Mechanisms

Both the pilot and then the full trial of Learning Together involved a comprehensive process evaluation. These included quantitative elements (focused on assessing intervention fidelity, reach and acceptability using surveys, provider diaries and tick-box observations by researchers) and qualitative elements (focused on providers' and recipients' views and experiences of the intervention using interviews and focus group discussions).[146][147]

We used qualitative research to examine mechanisms in two different ways.[148][149] The first approach is one suggested by realist evaluators.[150][151] This involves directly asking providers, recipients or other participants how they think an intervention works. Participants are asked what they think about the evaluators' starting CMOCs, to validate, refine or reject these. As Pawson (1996) comments:[150] '[T]he researcher's theory is the subject matter of the interview, and the subject is there to confirm or falsify and, above all, to refine that theory' (p. 299). Pawson further suggests that the interviewer should first 'teach' the participant about the starting theory of change and CMOCs before 'learning' from the participant which of these align with their experiences and how they might be refined:

> The subject's task is to agree, disagree and to categorize themselves in relation to the attitudinal patterns as constructed in [the researcher's] questions but also to refine their conceptual basis. It is at this point that mutual knowledge is really achieved. The subject is saying in effect 'this is how you have depicted the potential structure of my thinking, but in my experience it happened like this. (p. 306)

We used this technique to ask interview participants to consider our starting CMOCs and then comment on these or describe their own alternative theories. For example, one school student, trained as a conflict mediator as part of the intervention, responded to questions about how restorative practice works by describing how he thought this practice could resolve conflicts:

> I just thought [restorative practice] was a brilliant idea because it's showing the younger kids how to be mature about difficult situations and teaching them how to deal with it. And rather than just getting angry, sitting down and talking through things is a better solution. And it's just showing them that.
> (Focus group discussion with year 9 students, Meadowood School)

We did not conclude that any one participant's comments were, on their own, an authoritative guide to how the intervention worked. Instead, we used qualitative analysis methods to compare and contrast views expressed in different interviews and focus group discussions. This allowed us to understand how different participants were expressing the same ideas but in different words and to build up an overall picture of intervention mechanisms by drawing on multiple accounts. For example, our qualitative analyses suggested that where teachers felt they were able to implement the social and emotional skills curriculum, this could enable students to develop increased empathy and better negotiate conflict. Interviews and focus groups with students told a similar story. Students in one school described how they had learned to manage their emotions and social relationships constructively:

> I like the fact that we get ... that someone's actually teaching us how to control our emotions, so if there's an argument we know how to stop it. ... Instead of kicking off at your friends, just talk with a normal tone and just apologise and see how it goes from there.
> (Focus group with year 9 students, Meadowood School)

Interviews with staff at this school suggested that the process was contingent on teachers committing to deliver the curriculum as well as on students having deficits in social and emotional skills that the intervention could therefore usefully address. In another school, these deficits were felt not to be present so that the curriculum was perceived as less useful by staff. More generally, our process evaluation found that the social and emotional skills curriculum was in many schools not delivered with fidelity because teachers did not like some of the curriculum resources that the intervention provided.

We were cautious when using this direct approach to examining intervention mechanisms for two reasons. Firstly, it could be too abstract for some participants, particularly young people. Secondly, some participants might find it hard to disagree with researchers about how they thought an intervention worked, even when researchers' ideas do not reflect participants' experiences. This consideration is particularly important when conducting research with children, with whom there will always be a major power differential.

Our second approach to using qualitative research to refine CMOCs is less direct, focusing on participants' accounts of their own experiences rather than their views on our theories. In the case of Learning Together, we read through participants' accounts of how they were involved in enacting intervention processes, the conditions under which this occurred and the consequences that followed.[152] We identified recurring patterns of the conditions necessary for and the consequences arising from intervention activities. Partly this approach involves looking for regularities in what conditions seemed to us or to participants to be associated with particular actions, or in what consequences seemed to be associated with particular actions. But our analyses went beyond such quasi-quantitative assessment of conjunctions because they tried to pinpoint *exactly what it was about* certain conditions that seemed to enable certain actions to occur, or what it was about certain actions that allowed certain consequences to follow, an approach commonly used within qualitative research.[121] We explored how participants' accounts could shed light on our CMOCs, contradicting, elaborating or augmenting these. Any one participant might only comment on the actions involved in one subsection of a causal mechanism. However, as researchers, we could draw on several participants' accounts to develop a more comprehensive picture of these mechanisms, as described in previous empirical studies.[141] We then drew on these qualitative analyses to inform refinements to our CMOCs.

In the case of Learning Together, we used multiple interviews and focus groups to understand how the conditions present in action groups in some school contexts helped staff and students to develop mutual understanding and better relationships. For example, one student described becoming able to understand teachers' perspectives:

> I think mainly just having other people's, seeing other people's views and seeing how ... if we had the same views or ... hearing someone else's point of view and thinking, "Oh yeah."
> (Focus group with year 9 students, Meadowood School)

And interviews with other students suggested how developing empathy could improve relationships between students and teachers, which could increase students' commitment to working hard at school. As one student put it:

> If you have a bond with your teacher ... you want to do well for the teacher because you feel like she's paid attention to you and gave her respect [in action group meetings]. And the way you can respect her back is by working hard.
> (Focus group with year 8 students, St. Anselm's School)

However, it was clear that these processes only occurred, and indeed *could only occur*, in schools with action groups led by senior staff who believed in the intervention. Only such staff had the authority to make sure action groups were well-enough attended and well-enough run so that empathy could grow between staff and students in the course of well-run meetings. We could see how action groups could trigger mechanisms involving staff and students developing mutual empathy and students increasing their commitment to school but only in schools where senior staff ensured action groups ran well. Confidence in the plausibility of our CMOCs grew when we saw from the qualitative data that, in schools with less management capacity (e.g. only one staff member regularly attending meetings and students feeling like their input did not matter to the school leadership), students did not report that their relationships with staff or their commitment to school had improved.

It was also apparent from interviews in some schools that such mechanisms were also contingent on the intervention aligning with the school culture. In one academically selective school, the action group was, as we had hypothesised in our 'dark logic model', hijacked to orient the intervention towards promoting students' academic attainment more than their health. In some other schools characterised by an authoritarian ethos, the school signed up to the intervention but implementation was stymied by staff not really committing to the inclusive ethos of the intervention. No single participant proposed any of these theories or insights in their entirety. They were developed indirectly by piecing together insights from lots of different interviews and focus groups. It suggested to us that action groups could trigger mechanisms which built student empathy with staff and hence increased commitment to school but only in schools where organisational capacity and culture meant that action groups were well-enough run to trigger such mechanisms.

In another example, an interview focused on one student's experiences of restorative practice. The interview was with a boy who had encouraged his friend to take a photo of another boy on the toilet. This boy interviewed described how his sense of responsibility grew within the restorative practice meeting, and how the conditions present in this meeting enabled this:

> I normally would have been moaning [about being punished], saying "No" ... But this time I actually felt what I had done was really wrong. It just made me realise ... I mean it's ... just when I saw him sitting there in that state [crying during the meeting].
>
> (Interview with year 8 student, Harper's School)

We theorised that restorative practice could trigger a mechanism involving development of a sense of responsibility among perpetrators. Analysis of other interviews suggested that this would generate reductions in bullying but only when a critical mass of staff committed to delivering restorative practice and when there were sufficient incidents of bullying to ensure that it was commonly deployed. This is an example of how we used qualitative data to help us refine how we theorised mechanisms, incorporating the meaning intervention activities had for participants.[103][121] In the case of this second approach, we tried to approach the analysis of qualitative data with an open mind. Rather than directly refining our CMOCs through the analysis, we instead aimed to theorise intervention mechanisms and how these interact with context to generate outcomes. Only after we had completed the analysis did we use this to refine and develop new CMOCs.

Both the direct and the indirect approaches already described can be used in the same study or even the same interview. It has been suggested that initial exploratory interviews use the direct approach to help evaluators develop initial theories of how intervention activities might trigger mechanisms and the contextual contingencies affecting these. Later interviews can then consider and refine these theories.[151] This might often be useful, but this need not always be the order. Sometimes, qualitative research can start with the indirect approach, with interviews examining participants' accounts of how they were involved in enacting interventions, and the conditions for and consequences of this, before later interviews use the direct approach of explicitly discussing theories of change and CMOCs. It all depends on what is judged most appropriate with different participants and which interviews can practically speaking be scheduled first.

5.4 Sampling within Qualitative Research on Mechanisms

This brings us on to considering how we should sample sites and participants for participation in qualitative research aiming to contribute towards theory and CMOC refinement. Sampling should be purposive. It should seek to include diversity in terms of the characteristics of sites or individuals that we think might be important in the analysis. Usually this means thinking through what characteristics of sites or individuals are likely to be important in enabling us to include a diversity of different perspectives on the questions we are asking. In the trial of Learning Together, schools were selected as case study sites based on rates of student eligibility for free school meals and external facilitators' reports of the success of implementation. The former was a measure of student socio-economic status as a proxy indicator of the likely stresses that a school was under. The latter was a rough measure of how well the mechanisms were likely to have been triggered so we could get a sense of what factors affected this.

Within these case studies, we purposively sampled participants involved in different aspects of intervention delivery and receipt, including students, school leaders, classroom teachers, intervention developers and external facilitators. These different people were likely to have interesting and diverse perspectives on how the intervention was delivered and how this might or might not have impacted on schools. Within the student groups, we sought further diversity by interviewing students who had bullied or had been bullied, as well as those who had or had not participated in Learning Together activities, as these students would likely have different experiences. Moreover, bullying tends to be a highly gendered activity, so being deliberate about trying to speak to a gender diverse group of students allowed us to assess how gender was relevant to the various mechanisms activated and under what contexts. It is also a good idea for qualitative research to have some flexibility in sampling sites and individuals so that, if initial analyses suggest different mechanisms or interactions with context than initially theorised, these can be further explored with appropriate sites and participants. This variation of purposive sampling is described by some qualitative analysts as 'theoretical sampling', because ongoing sampling is based on seeking out the kinds of experiences we need to test and refine our developing theory.

A key question for sampling in a realist evaluation is whose accounts are going to be most informative when examining different aspects of intervention mechanisms. Ana Manzano has suggested that provider managers will have a broad overview of patterns of successes and failures and so will provide authoritative information on how mechanisms are contingent on context. She suggests that practitioners will probably be able to provide further detail about the specific conditions affecting mechanisms locally. And she adds that clients will be able to describe their personal experiences of impacts but may have less to say about mechanisms or how these interact with context.[151] This was not our experience with the Learning Together process evaluation. We found that school leaders and external facilitators often focused on implementation of intervention activities rather than the mechanisms that these might trigger. They also tended to present the 'official' theory of change, telling us what they thought we wanted to hear. Students and classroom teachers often had much more to say about what mechanisms might have been triggered and how these might have interacted with context to generate reductions in bullying. For example, the student accounts quoted in Section 5.3 were useful in exploring the consequences of participation in restorative practice.

5.5 Qualitative Data Collection

Let us turn now to how to run interviews and focus group discussions. These involve open-ended questions allowing the participants to describe their experiences and views in their own words. They should take the form of a conversation rather than an interrogation. Interviewers should take care not to offer too many of their own views and ensure that interviewees get a chance to express their views. Sessions are normally structured using a guide with a list of general topics rather than a list of prescriptive questions. The order with which topics are addressed may vary so that the participant's story is followed and prioritised. What matters is that all the topics are addressed rather than exactly how questions are worded or ordered. Interviews and focus groups can take a direct approach, exploring participants' views on theories of change, or an indirect approach, understanding the conditions and consequences of participants' actions. When using the direct approach, the researcher will tend to control the interview process more tightly, asking focused questions about mechanisms. Manzano gives the following examples:[151]

> For example: 'How was your work different before the programme was implemented?', 'Is this new programme going to work for everyone?', 'Could you explain to me the types of people and places where you think it may be more effective?' Stronger questions about context should encourage people to compare subgroups, location, times, before and after. The objective is to draw the interviewee into comparison to explore contextual effectiveness. (pp. 354–5)

In the case of the less direct approach, the interview or focus group will be more participant centred, exploring participants' experiences. The interviewer may use prompts to explore how the participants' actions were influenced by intervention resources and activities, local policies or norms or the presence of economic or other resources.[103] In the case of Learning Together, interviews with those who had taken part in action groups explored how group activities were enabled or constrained by the intervention manual, external facilitator and training, as well as the broader management structure, priorities, culture and resourcing of the school. Interviews explored the consequences the action groups had for how the school operated, and how students and staff acted and interacted.

5.6 Qualitative Data Analysis

Once the data have been collected, they need to be analysed. Existing literature offers some pointers on how this should be done. Realist evaluators have suggested, for example, that qualitative data should be coded in terms of '"description of the actual intervention", "observed outcomes", "context conditions" and "underlying mechanisms"' (p. 195) to inform refinement of CMOCs.[117] But existing literature doesn't offer comprehensive guidance on analysis. A useful place to start is by recognising that participant accounts are themselves an interpretation of their experiences of reality so that any analysis of such accounts involves a 'double hermeneutic' (i.e. an interpretation of an interpretation).[116][153] This does not mean that qualitative research shouldn't aim to shed light on the underlying reality.[153] But it does mean that any experience which interviewees report is mediated by their own interpretations. This is a strength, not a weakness, of qualitative research because how participants understand an intervention and its consequences will likely be central to its mechanism.[153] For example, within the evaluation of the Learning Together intervention, our analyses explored how staff and students emphasised the intervention's participative nature, which participants often associated with its ability to transform relationships within their school:

> I think that the students will certainly enjoy the fact that we're doing something like this so they can be involved in it and that they can actually have their voice heard, that they can feel safe at school, that they can feel engaged with the teachers, that they can feel they're listened to.   (Staff, Harper's School, staff interview)

Qualitative analysis aims ultimately to inform refinement of the theory of change and CMOCs. In the Learning Together process evaluation, we put aside our existing theory of change and CMOCs as we analysed our qualitative data. We did this so that we could make full use of our qualitative data and so our analysis was not driven by our starting theories. We then used the resulting analyses to refine our CMOCs.

To help inform theorisation of mechanisms, analyses should do more than merely identify recurring themes. Within realist evaluation, analysis will need to explore how mechanisms seem to interact with context to generate outcomes. Qualitative research needs to be orientated towards theory building to do this. In the Learning Together evaluation, we used an analytical method based on 'grounded theory'. Grounded theory is an approach to qualitative analysis which aims to build theory from analysis of social processes.[154] A hallmark of grounded theory is the analytic method known as *constant comparison*, which focuses on comparing different data within and between interviewee accounts against each other from the very start and throughout the analytic process, with the goal of developing new ideas to be tested and refined as sampling progresses. We used a variant of grounded theory called 'dimensional analysis'.[152] This offers a framework for building theory about social phenomena in terms of their broad *context* (the boundaries of a phenomenon), *conditions* (the specific factors facilitating, blocking or otherwise influencing social actions associated with a phenomenon), *process* (the actions or interactions involved in a phenomenon), *consequences* (what happens as a result of these actions) and *outcomes* (changes in people as a result of the phenomenon).

While the language is slightly different, these broad constructs map onto realist CMOCs. It is important to note that what, in dimensional analysis, we would call 'conditions' are what realists generally mean when they discuss 'context'. Within dimensional analysis, 'context' is broader and will include phenomena that are experienced across all sites and participants, which may contribute to generating outcomes but will not be specific only to some sites. What is called 'process' in dimensional analysis can be used to encompass the interactional aspects of 'mechanisms' as defined within realist evaluation. What are called 'consequences' in dimensional analysis align with what are referred to as 'outcomes' in realist evaluation. We can also tie together different CMOCs into a *perspective*, which refers to a broader theme with sufficient explanatory power to make sense of the CMOCs.

We thought dimensional analysis would be a good approach to use to develop grounded theory about how intervention mechanisms interact with context to generate outcomes. Grounded theory methods and dimensional analysis were developed within what is known as the 'symbolic interactionist' approach to sociology (which tries to understand how our understandings of the world are built from social interactions and communication).[155] While realism does not share this focus, this does not mean that grounded theory or dimensional analysis are incompatible with realist approaches to understanding social phenomena, including realist evaluation. Grounded theory approaches have previously been used within realist evaluation.[154 156 157]

In the Learning Together study, we used dimensional analysis to analyse interview and focus group transcripts.[149] We coded these according to whether they described or implied *process* (e.g. interactions between staff and students, encouraging students to increase their commitment to school), linked within or across interviews to accounts of *conditions* (e.g. students or staff having positive experiences of participating in the action group) and *consequences* (e.g. decreasing student involvement in anti-school peer groups).

Our understanding of mechanisms needs to start from the point at which they are triggered by the use of intervention resources in specific contexts all the way through to how these mechanisms generate outcomes. Because everyone's perspective is partial, no one participant will have a panoramic perspective on the full mechanism. As a result, our analyses will usually need to draw on multiple accounts across different interviews and/or focus groups to theorise mechanisms from start to finish. In the Learning Together process evaluation, for example, we developed theory as to how enactment of action groups might trigger mechanisms which generate student commitment and which ultimately generate reductions in student aggression. This theorisation was pieced together from insights garnered from many different accounts. A teacher would comment on how involvement in action groups could increase student commitment to school. A student would comment on how increased commitment to school might lead them to be more prepared to follow school rules and not bully other students. Consistent with our grounded theory approach, our analyses had to compare and contrast different accounts, deciding as we went which accounts provide more or less authoritative insights into particular sections of the mechanism.

As well as understanding mechanisms, qualitative analyses need to explore the conditions necessary for mechanisms to 'trigger'. Such analyses might start by examining patterns of contingencies (e.g. if this condition was present, then this consequence usually seemed to follow). But, as argued in Section 5.3, these analyses should go beyond this to explore *exactly what it is about* the conditions that enable certain actions, or *what is it about* certain actions that generate certain consequences.[121] These analyses can use specific techniques from grounded theory to do this, such as trying to explain deviant cases. Deviant cases refer to data that can't be explained by the analysis as it currently stands. The analysis needs to be refined so that it can explain these deviant cases.[93] For example, some of our insights into what conditions were necessary to ensure action groups could trigger mechanisms generating increased student commitment came from interviews in a school where the action group did not attract broad staff involvement and so failed to encourage staff and students to understand each other better.

5.7 The Status of Theory Built through Qualitative Research

Through these different approaches, qualitative research can build theory about how intervention mechanisms might interact with context to generate outcomes. This can then be compared with starting theory or CMOCs to decide how these need to be refined.

However, it is important to recognise that any such theories or CMOCs, even if refined through qualitative research, might still be wrong. This is a point on which we disagree with critical realist social scientists, such as Andrew Sayer, who have argued that only qualitative research can provide a valid consideration of social mechanisms.[121] We have several reasons for arguing that theory built through qualitative research should then be tested using quantitative research. Firstly, qualitative analyses will be limited by the fallibility of participants' own accounts.[121] Many people will not be all that interested in identifying the conditions which affected their actions or the consequences of their actions and, even if they are, their perceptions might not be correct. This will be particularly the case for the more 'upstream' conditions or the more 'downstream' consequences of actions. Drawing on multiple accounts will help here but will only partially compensate for these limitations. Qualitative research is strong on understanding meaning rather than cause and effect. Secondly, qualitative research will draw on a limited sample of sites and participants. Qualitative research aims to develop valid conclusions not by the statistical representativeness of its samples but rather by encompassing diverse accounts and deep analysis to develop nuanced theory. But even so, samples are usually small and so can miss important experiences or views that might change the analysis.[158] In practice, saturation is rarely achieved.

This means that what qualitative research provides is a way to refine our theories and CMOCs rather than a means to arrive at fully validated conclusions about cause and effect. To examine the latter, our theories and CMOCs need to be tested using some of the various statistical analysis methods described in the next chapter. Some mechanisms that we theorise will be just too complex to subject to quantitative analysis. They might involve complex cycles of positive feedback for example. In such cases, quantitative research might be able to focus on testing some but not all aspects of mechanisms and, for other aspects, qualitative research may be as far as the analysis can go. Some mechanisms might, in principle, be open to quantitative testing but be developed at a point in an evaluation when it is too late to include suitable quantitative measures in our questionnaires. In such cases, these hypotheses might need to be examined in future studies. These limitations should be documented and suggestions for further investigations noted in any publications or reports that emerge from the evaluation.

In Box 5.1, we summarise the CMOCs refined through the qualitative research.

5.8 Qualitative Research on Mechanisms during Different Evaluation Phases

Feasibility and Pilot Studies

Now that we have described our general approach to using qualitative research within process evaluations to inform refinement of intervention theory of change and CMOCs, let us consider how this might come into play at the pilot or feasibility stage, and at the effectiveness trial phase.

Analysis of data from process evaluations conducted within feasibility or pilot studies can provide early information about the plausibility of CMOCs. Feasibility and pilot studies are designed as initial checks on intervention feasibility and acceptability before investing more time and resources into expensive studies of effectiveness. Although the difference between feasibility and pilot studies is debated,[159] the term 'pilot study' usually refers to

Box 5.1 Summary of refinement of Learning Together CMOCs informed by qualitative research conducted in the process evaluation

'Sense of Belonging' Mechanism of Benefit

Context: Particularly among socio-economically disadvantaged students, and in schools with strong organisational capacity and an inclusive culture which enables effective and inclusive action groups.

Mechanism: The action group enables reclassification and reframing in schools so that boundaries between staff and students are eroded, students feel they have made a positive contribution and mutual empathy is engendered.

Outcome: Generating increased student sense of belonging in school, increased commitment to school social norms and reductions in bullying.

'Perpetration Curtailment' Mechanism of Benefit

Context: Particularly in schools where a critical mass of staff committed to delivering restorative practice and there were sufficient incidents of bullying to ensure that it was commonly deployed.

Mechanism: Restorative practice enables perpetrators to develop responsibility for actions and empathy with victims.

Outcome: Generating curtailment of bullying perpetration.

'Social and Emotional Skills' Mechanism of Benefit

Context: Particularly in schools where staff commit to delivering these components and where student deficits in social and emotional skills are critical to mechanisms generating bullying.

Mechanism: The classroom curriculum and/or the preventative use of restorative practice enable students to develop social and emotional skills.

Outcome: Generating avoidance of conflict and reductions in bullying.

'Hijacking' Mechanism of Harm

There was qualitative evidence for this mechanism but only in a small number of academically selective schools.

'Labelling' Mechanism of Harm

There was no evidence for this mechanism.

'Disruption' Mechanism of Harm

There was no evidence for this mechanism.

---

a miniature version of the main trial. These include implementation of the intervention and the piloting of the evaluation methods, though in fewer sites, with fewer participants and/or for a shorter period than would be the case in the planned main study of effectiveness. In contrast, the term 'feasibility study' is used to refer to a study focusing only on select aspects of an intervention or evaluation about which there are uncertainties. Following the development of MRC guidance on complex interventions,[39][160] the number of feasibility and pilot studies, particularly pilot RCTs, has rapidly increased.[159]

These studies are very useful from a realist perspective. Refinements can be made to the intervention (and to its theory of change and CMOCs) after a pilot or feasibility study. In an effectiveness trial, we can refine the theory of change and CMOCs but we can't refine the intervention itself. Modifying an intervention midway through an effectiveness trial would muddy the water too much as to what intervention was being evaluated and therefore what intervention might be scaled up should the trial report that the interventions were effective. For this reason, the process evaluation in an effectiveness trial is usually separately managed from the management of the intervention so that results from the former cannot influence the latter.

Realist analysis within feasibility and pilot studies should explore implementation and possible mechanisms in a range of contexts prior to larger effectiveness trials. Such preliminary studies provide an opportunity to examine potential barriers and facilitators to implementation in a range of settings; to explore the views of those involved and assess how these vary by different contexts; and to refine and optimise the intervention design, logic model and trial methods. However, to date, most feasibility studies and pilot trials have only answered relatively crude, binary questions about whether a specific complex intervention is feasible and acceptable, or not. They have rarely examined how mechanisms might interact with context to generate outcomes. This is a missed opportunity. The dominance of binary assessments of feasibility is reflected in the widespread use of binary 'progression criteria' to determine whether a subsequent, larger evaluation is justified. Progression criteria stipulate whether, for example, an intervention has been delivered with a certain level of fidelity, reach or acceptability. Feasibility and pilot studies should also assess what is feasible and acceptable for whom and under what conditions, aiming to refine theory of change and CMOCs, and, if necessary, intervention resources and methods. Several realist strategies could be used at this stage.

First, purposive sampling criteria should be used in feasibility and pilot studies to ensure these encompass sufficient diversity in aspects of context pre-hypothesised to influence feasibility, acceptability and/or causal mechanisms. Our pilot trial of Learning Together used a purposive sampling matrix to recruit a theoretically informed diversity of schools that varied according to the socio-economic status of their students (measured by rates of student free school meal eligibility) and organisational capacity (measured by national inspectorate ratings of school 'effectiveness'). The study also purposively sampled a range of staff and students varying respectively by role/seniority and socio-demographic characteristics.[161]

Second, as is the case with subsequent effectiveness trials, feasibility and pilot trials enable the collection and analysis of qualitative data to support the refinement of theories of change and CMOCs. They do not aim to estimate intervention effects, so research teams can collect much more data (especially qualitative data) from intervention or control groups without worrying about the impact of evaluation activities on study outcomes, confounding estimates of intervention effects.[162] Therefore, these preliminary studies are where the heavy lifting of CMOC refinement should ideally occur. Some of the progression criteria set for a feasibility or pilot study could focus on whether CMOCs have been refined based on the study.

Effectiveness Studies

Studies powered to assess intervention effectiveness (sometimes called 'phase III studies') should not just assess effectiveness. Process evaluations conducted within such studies provide a means of refining CMOCs prior to their being tested using quantitative outcome data. Process evaluations within trials aim to provide a check that interventions were delivered and received as planned. This may be important, for example, in interpreting null effects from outcome evaluations, so that researchers can determine whether any limitations in effectiveness reflect a real lack of validity of the theory of change (as applied to the context) or merely a failure of implementation. Process evaluations also enable us to better understand how intervention feasibility and acceptability vary and what factors influence this. Effectiveness studies are larger and inevitably more diverse than feasibility or pilot studies in the contexts they include, and this enables us to get a better sense of what contextual factors will influence implementation. Unpicking this will inform later judgements about to which settings interventions might most appropriately be transferred.

Qualitative and quantitative data from process evaluations can be used to shed light on whether our CMOCs are plausible and, if not, how they might be refined. Again, the greater diversity of contexts within effectiveness studies aids such analyses. However, with the collection of evaluation data, the risk arises that evaluation activities exert their own effects which might be detected in follow-up assessments, introducing confounding into our estimates of intervention effects. It might be, for example, that participating in such a detailed process evaluation has direct effects on measures of our outcomes. Or participation in evaluation activities might generate resentment or too much work for staff who then disengage from delivering the intervention. For this reason, it is preferable for most of the examination of mechanisms to occur within pilot and feasibility studies. However, it is usually the case that evaluators want to continue to use process evaluations to examine implementation and explore mechanisms in trials of effectiveness. Where this is the case, it is a good idea to try to minimise biases arising from the impacts of evaluation activities by trying to ensure that these are as light touch as possible, and occur as equally as possible in both intervention and control arms. The testing of CMOCs within effectiveness trials is the subject of the next chapter.

Chapter 6

Testing Realist Theory through Trials or Other Evaluation Designs

This chapter is about how we can use quantitative analyses within trials to test CMOCs and therefore better understand how mechanisms interact with context to generate outcomes. We believe that there is an important role for such analyses in checking whether the patterns and regularities we find in quantitative data appear to align with what we would predict based on our theories of how interventions work, for whom and under what circumstances. This is a controversial area. Some realist evaluators support the use of quantitative alongside qualitative data to shed light on mechanisms.[117] Indeed, the originators of realist evaluators, Pawson and Tilley, argue that they are 'methods neutral'. Other realist evaluators and many other critical realist researchers are strongly opposed to using quantitative methods. They argue that explanation of causation in the social world should not be reduced to the search for 'constant conjunctions'. Andrew Sayer, for example, has argued that quantitative research fails to recognise that in 'open systems' (e.g. the institutions or communities in which interventions are delivered and trials are conducted) these regularities rarely occur:[121]

> [E]vents arise from the workings of mechanisms which derived from the structures of objects, and they take place within geo-historical contexts. This contrasts with approaches which treat the world as if it were no more than patterns of events, to be registered by recording punctiform data regarding 'variables' and looking for regularities among them. ... Given the variety and changeability of the contexts of social life, this absence of regular associations between 'causes' and 'effects' should be expected. (pp. 15–16)

We recognise this risk but we do think it is often informative to explore regularities quantitatively. This applies not just to evaluations but also to health and social research more generally. Obvious examples of where there *are* empirical regularities which *do* shed light on important social mechanisms include that people in nations with high levels of income inequality generally experience worse health outcomes (affecting all social classes) than those in countries with lower levels of income inequality;[163] within countries, those of lower socio-economic status tend to experience worse health than those of higher socio-economic status;[164] and schools which engage all students in learning generally have lower rates of student violence and substance use.[132]

In Chapter 3, we outlined why we disagreed with the criticism that trials inappropriately use a 'successionist' approach. Our argument applies to quantitative research more generally. We argued that using statistical analyses to identify associations between variables actually recognises that conjunctions are not constant. If they were constant in the sense of always being present, then the value of statistical measures of association (such as odds ratios) would be zero or infinity. Statistical assessment of associations measures *tendencies*

51

towards association rather than all or nothing conjunctions. For example, if a trial were to report a 30 per cent reduction in bullying, that would not mean that each individual's experience with bullying was 30 per cent lessened but rather that, for an overall population, 30 per cent fewer people were affected than normal. We also explained how statistical analyses can look at more nuanced patterns of association. For example, moderation analyses can examine how the association between two variables is contingent on the presence of a third. We also explained how analyses of quantitative variables from the realm of the empirical does not mean that one cannot draw on these to test and refine deeper theory about how mechanisms interact with context in the realm of the real to generate outcomes.

In this chapter, we aim to show how CMOCs refined using qualitative research within process evaluations can then be tested using quantitative data within trials or other quantitative-based study designs. We first describe what a 'realist trial' needs to look like if it is to enable such testing. The term 'realist RCT' refers to a large, mixed method trial that combines the advantages of minimising bias in effect estimates and other analyses (by employing randomisation and all the other useful features of trials that we described in Chapter 2) with the ability to refine and test hypotheses about CMOCs as described in Chapters 3–5.[165] [166] Guidance from the United Kingdom's Medical Research Council supports this combination of features within trials.[1] [2]

So, what are the features of a realist trial? To be able to test CMOCs, trials need to recruit and retain a sufficiently diverse sample of sites and populations in terms of the characteristics that are referred to in their starting CMOCs. For example, if a CMOC refers to context in terms of individuals' socio-economic status or the extent to which sites are urban or rural, then the trial needs to ensure that its inclusion criteria and sampling methods allow for inclusion of urban and rural sites as well as individuals of different socio-economic statuses. Although some realist evaluators are convinced that this is impossible,[37] we see no reason why it should be. There are no insurmountable barriers to achieving this.

In the trial of Learning Together, our sample included a diversity of schools and of students, which broadly reflected the profile of schools and students in England.[125] Our schools were representative in terms of size, population demographic factors, deprivation and educational performance, but were slightly more likely to have a positive government inspection rating. When we randomised schools to intervention or control group, we used a method called 'stratification' to ensure that the two groups were balanced according to single-sex versus mixed-sex schools, school-level socio-economic deprivation and student examination attainment. We did this by grouping schools according to these factors and then randomising within these groups. This ensured that the trial arms were balanced according to these factors. The 'control' that stratification exerted did not aim to reduce the diversity of schools or students in our trial. Rather, it simply aimed to ensure that there was a similar *degree* of diversity in each arm. This meant that our sample was diverse enough to allow us to explore how these aspects of context (in terms of setting and population) might influence how outcomes were generated while still enabling us to estimate the extent to which bullying was reduced compared to usual practice. Other trials have successfully aimed to encompass diversity in various other theoretically important contextual factors.[114] [167]

Realist trials also need to have a long enough follow-up period so that the theorised mechanisms have enough time to generate outcomes. They should also, where possible, include an intermediate follow-up before the final one. This allows for the measurement of potential mediator variables before the measurement of 'end' outcomes. For example, the trial of Learning Together had a final follow-up survey three years after our baseline surveys. This period was chosen, informed by previous research,[168] as the one likely to be the time needed for our theorised mechanisms of school organisational change enabling the generation of beneficial impacts for students. An intermediate follow-up occurred after two years to assess mediators. We judged this long enough for the generation of these intermediate outcomes informed by previous research.[168]

Realist trials need to include quantitative measures that will shed light on the contexts, mechanisms and outcomes referred to in the theory of change and CMOCs. Using such quantitative measures doesn't mean that we think that these aspects of the realm of the real can be reduced to these variables in the realm of the empirical. But quantitative analysis of these measures can provide indirect insights into how these mechanisms operate in the realm of the real. Outcome analyses assess whether allocation of people or clusters of people to an intervention is associated with more reporting of a beneficial outcome (e.g. mental well-being) or less reporting of an adverse outcome (e.g. bullying victimisation) among the intervention group compared to the control group. Outcome variables are measured at the final follow-up.

We can then use moderation and mediation analyses to unpack overall effects. These two terms are often confused, but they mean very different things. Moderation analyses assess whether the association between two variables is dependent on a third, the moderator. For example, they might assess whether the association between allocations to an intervention with an outcome is contingent on a certain participant or cluster characteristic. Moderator variables are measured at baseline and examine context in terms of descriptors of subgroups of settings or populations. Traditionally, in trials, moderators examine factors such as participants' gender or sex, age, socio-economic status or ethnicity, for example, to assess intervention effects on health inequalities. Analysing whether interventions have differential effectiveness by subgroups can suggest where equity harms or benefits are in evidence. Such factors may still be what is examined in moderator analysis within realist trials, but realist trials might measure other, more theoretically informed aspects of context too, informed by CMOCs. For example, in our trial of Learning Together we wanted to see whether intervention effects were moderated by factors such as school baseline organisational capacity.

Mediation analyses, on the other hand, assess whether the association between two variables can be accounted for by the presence of a third intervening variable, the mediator, which is generally an intermediate outcome of the intervention. Mediator variables are best measured at interim follow-up (also called mid-line). This permits what is called a 'fully longitudinal mediation analysis', where the intervention (which is allocated at baseline) causes a change in the mediator (which is measured at interim follow-up), which then precedes the measurement of the final outcome (which is measured at final follow-up). This fully longitudinal model increases our confidence that change in the mediator brought about by the intervention in fact precedes change in the final outcome. Therefore, in realist trials, mediation analysis can be used to explore the impact of mechanisms.

Like traditional randomised trials, realist trials also need to be adequately powered. In other words, they must have big enough samples to allow us to answer our research questions. Because realist trials are focused not merely on the overall effects of an intervention but also on whether these effects vary with context, they need to employ bigger than normal samples. Moderation analyses require larger sample sizes, especially where some subgroups characterised by a moderator variable (e.g. LGBTQ+ identity in a school trial) are smaller than others. Most trials are currently powered on the basis of detecting overall intervention effects on a primary outcome, so that moderator analyses are often underpowered.[169] The analyses can still be run even when the sample is too small, but they may fail to detect moderation that actually is present but is too subtle to be detected in too small a study. This is currently the most significant barrier to testing CMOCs within trials. However, even where a single trial lacks the power for such analyses, all is not lost. Reporting the results of such underpowered analyses is still useful because it then allows for these to be included within systematic reviews and meta-analyses oriented towards realist questions (see Chapter 8). To facilitate this, different trials focused on similar interventions, populations and outcomes should as far as possible use similar measures so that they can be put together in systematic reviews. We consider this question in more detail in Chapter 8.

Realist trials should also be guided by protocols, but these need to be updated to account for the refining of theory and CMOCs that occurs during process evaluations integral to them. We saw in Chapter 2 that the conduct and reporting of trials must be guided by protocols that are registered and publicly available. Crucially, this ensures that trial reports are transparent about which analyses were pre-planned and which were post hoc. This ensures that evaluators, or those who fund them, cannot switch outcome measures from those originally intended to other measures when the latter but not the former show evidence of significant benefits from the intervention. This practice is known as 'data dredging' and can be a major source of 'publication bias' where protocols are not enforced. Unlike conventional trials, realist trials refine their hypotheses in the course of the study. We described in the previous chapter the process by which this happens.

In order to retain the advantages of a protocol for probity, while allowing refinement of CMOCs so that the statistical analyses test the most plausible hypotheses, realist trials should use 'living protocols'.[126] An initial protocol should be publicly registered as it would be for a conventional trial, with inclusion of any planned mediation and moderation analyses to test CMOCs. Updates should then be posted on the registration site to indicate how the CMOCs have been refined in the course of the study and how this will change the trial analyses. In order to preserve public and policy confidence in such trials, overall primary and secondary outcome analyses should not change, but moderator and mediator analyses can change.

6.1 Incorporating Realist Evaluation into Non-randomised Evaluations

Randomised trials are the strongest design to estimate overall intervention effects and to test CMOCs using quantitative data. Crucially, randomisation is the best means we have to ensure fair comparisons and minimise bias and confounding in our statistical analyses. However, as we reported in Chapter 2, sometimes there are practical challenges to conducting randomised trials. We think that, given the advantages of randomisation, ways of surmounting these challenges should be carefully considered so that a randomised trial is used where it is appropriate. For example, where there is clear uncertainty about intervention benefits, it may be possible to persuade intervention providers and potential recipients that evaluation is required and that a randomised trial is ethical. Expert practitioners might be persuaded that they should have a role in determining which individuals (or clusters) are suitable candidates for an intervention but that random allocation should then be used to decide who within this pool gets the intervention and who is a control.[22] In some cases, 'client choice' can be accommodated in 'preference trials'. These allow clients to opt for random allocation or choose their preferred intervention.[170] Professional, policy or community advocates of a particular intervention may be persuaded that stepped-wedge or crossover trials are more acceptable. Stepped-wedge trials randomly allocate not whether individuals or clusters receive an intervention at all but instead randomise when they will receive it.[171] In crossover trials, all participants or clusters receive the intervention for a period and the control condition for a period. Randomisation determines the order in which this happens. In both cases, these designs can raise practical challenges and may not be suitable for evaluating interventions where it is expected that outcomes will take some time to manifest.[172]

However, in some cases, randomised controlled trials are simply not possible. This is not a reason to give up trying to evaluate interventions involved or allow a race to the bottom as to what design is used in the evaluation. In such cases, the best must not be the enemy of the good and we must simply find the next best way to evaluate the intervention. When random allocation is not possible, it may still be possible to employ a non-randomised control group. Such studies are often termed 'quasi-experimental studies'. There is a risk with such designs that the intervention and control groups will differ from one another at baseline in relation to factors that will influence the outcomes of interest and will therefore not be a fair comparison. This risk can be reduced but not eliminated by matching or weighting the control and intervention groups to each other, focusing on factors known to influence the outcome(s) in question. Statistical analyses can also be used to adjust for any known and measured baseline differences to further improve the fairness of the comparison. None of these methods is perfect because they can only account for potential confounders that are known about and measured. Other, fancier approaches can sometimes be used to make for a fair comparison, such as propensity score matching or instrumental variables. We will not discuss these further here but suffice to say neither of these offers a magic way of overcoming the risk of unfair comparisons.[173]

When it is not even possible to recruit a prospective control group, it may instead be possible to compare outcomes in the intervention group with rates in the general population. This approach has been used, for example, in studies evaluating the effects of new roads on mortality and injuries.[174] If rates change in the intervention group but not in the general population, this provides some evidence for intervention effects, though, again, these estimates may be liable to confounding as well as to regression to the mean, which we described in Chapter 2.[172]

In the absence of any external comparison, the next best design is a 'before-and-after' study in which outcomes are simply compared to baselines among an intervention group. Such studies are, of course, vulnerable to mistaking a change in outcomes caused by regression to the mean, secular or maturational trends or a specific other event for a change caused by the intervention. How much these undermine an evaluation will depend on context. Secular trends are less of a problem where rates of an outcome are stable within a population. Maturational trends are more of a problem with child and adolescent than adult populations.[172]

Sometimes not even comparison with baselines is possible. In such cases, all that can be done is to assess post-intervention measures of outcomes with post-intervention measures of exposure to the outcome. This was, for example, the case in an evaluation of the impact of a family planning intervention in Nepal, which used a radio soap opera to promote the concept of a 'well-planned family' and increase demand for contraception.[175] Such a design is weaker than one involving a control group or comparing outcomes with baselines because it usually relies on the assessment of exposure to the intervention via self-reports. This might bias an evaluation because those who report experiencing an outcome might be more likely to remember being exposed to the intervention.

All of these alternative designs will provide weaker evidence of causality because they are more likely to involve unfair comparisons. For this reason, they will also provide weaker evidence testing CMOCs. Nonetheless, where there is no alternative but to use such designs and where evaluators want to understand how mechanisms interact with context to generate outcomes, these designs can still incorporate realist design elements. They should, where possible, encompass sufficient diversity in their recruited sites and populations so that CMOCs can be tested; have long enough time between intervention and measurement of outcomes so that the theorised mechanisms have enough time to generate outcomes; include an intermediate follow-up before the final one to assess mediators (not possible of course in cross-sectional studies); include quantitative measures that will shed light on contexts, mechanisms and outcomes (possible even in cross-sectional studies although the temporal relationships between these may be unclear); include large enough samples so that moderation can be examined; and be guided by living protocols that can account for refined CMOCs and therefore modified study hypotheses. Furthermore, such evaluations should examine properly theorised interventions and include qualitative research within process evaluations so that theories of change are explicit and CMOCs are developed and open to refinement.

6.2 Quantitative Analyses to Shed Light on Context–Mechanism–Outcome Configurations

Now that we have described the key design elements of a realist trial or other quantitative evaluation, let us consider what analyses should be conducted within such trials using quantitative data to test CMOC hypotheses.

Overall Effect Analyses

As we argued in Chapter 3, realist trials should still report an intervention's overall effects because this may be evidence that policymakers need to assess the overall value of an intervention. This is particularly the case for preventive public health interventions for which population-level impacts are important.[85] In the case of Learning Together, the trial's overall analysis of primary outcomes was done using an intention to treat approach as explained in Chapter 2. This analysis reported a significant impact on students' self-reported bullying victimisation at thirty-six-month follow-up but no effects on perpetration of aggressive behaviours.[125] Regarding secondary outcomes, the intervention was associated with benefits in terms of increased health-related quality of life and mental well-being, and reduced psychological difficulties, smoking tobacco, drinking alcohol and illicit drug use. Subsequent exploratory analyses also found intervention effects on reduced e-cigarette use, cyberbullying perpetration, perpetration of aggressive behaviours, participation in school disciplinary procedures and truancy.[176] A separately funded analysis that used administrative data on students' performance in public examinations linked to trial data also found an intervention effect on improved academic attainment.[177] We also conducted some latent transition analyses to examine how the intervention appeared to act at the individual level to move students between different categories from baseline to follow-up.[178] This found that the intervention had a significant impact moving those students who were heavily involved in perpetration of aggressive behaviours at baseline into no or lower levels of aggression at follow-up.[179]

Moderation Analyses

Moderator analyses divide the sample into subgroups based on the moderator variable (e.g. high and low socio-economic status) and then assess whether the intervention's effect on the outcome is significantly different between these subgroups. This is sometimes referred to as interaction or effect modification.[180] These can be informative in trials. One use is in examining the impacts of interventions on health inequalities.[181] Another use, which is our focus in this book, is on understanding how intervention mechanisms might interact with context to generate outcomes. For example, an evaluation of a Welsh intervention to refer healthcare patients for physical exercise[182] involved moderation analyses examining how intervention effects varied by subgroup. It reported that the programme did not increase physical activity for those patients referred because of their mental health but did increase this for those referred because of their risk of coronary heart disease.[182] A trial of an intervention improving the way in which healthy options in university canteens were marketed to students was effective in improving students' intake of vegetables, but particularly so in those canteens which offered the highest quality dishes.[183]

In the Learning Together trial, our initial moderator analyses were primarily done to describe intervention effects on health inequalities rather than to investigate our CMOCs. However, these analyses found that intervention effects on bullying victimisation were no greater (or smaller) among students of low socio-economic status. This ran counter to our theory of change and initial CMOCs, which postulated that the intervention would have greater benefits for more socio-economically disadvantaged students. Other subgroup analyses reported that the intervention was more effective in preventing bullying victimisation for boys, and for students who at baseline reported previously being bullied and perpetrating aggressive behaviour. These analyses were interesting and important in understanding how and for whom the intervention worked, but did not shed light on our existing CMOCs.

Mediation Analyses

Mediation analyses can be useful in realist studies by assessing whether the effects of an intervention on an outcome can be accounted for by the effect of the intervention on an intermediate outcome. Such analyses don't examine how effects vary for different participants or sites but they do tell us something about how intervention mechanisms might work. In the Learning Together trial, we analysed whether intervention effects on the prevention of bullying victimisation were mediated by changes to how schools were organised, student commitment to school and student involvement in anti-school peer groups. These analyses did not test CMOCs because they did not attend to questions of how mechanisms might differ by context. But they did aim to throw some light on whether our theories about the mechanisms generating outcomes were correct. Our measure of school organisation examined the extent to which schools eroded boundaries between staff and students, students' academic and personal development and schools and their local communities.[184] Our measure of student commitment examined whether students felt positively about school in terms of academic engagement, sense of belonging, sense of participation and relationships with teachers.[185] Our measure of involvement in anti-school peer groups assessed whether students' friends had been in trouble with the police.[11] We hypothesised that intervention effects on bullying victimisation after three years of follow-up would be mediated by these measures of school organisation, student commitment and students' involvement in anti-school peer groups, all measured after two years of follow-up.

Mediation analyses can be undertaken in several ways. In this analysis, we used a method described as 'causal steps'.[186][187] Applied to trials, the first step looks at whether the intervention has an impact on the end outcome. We have already reported this in the section titled 'Overall Effects Analyses' – it did. The next step is to see whether the intervention has an impact on the mediator. The final step is to see whether including the mediator in a statistical model looking at the association between the intervention and the end outcome (in this case, bullying victimisation) causes the association between intervention and end outcome to reduce. A reduction indicates that at least some of the pathway from the intervention to the end outcome is explained by a route involving the mediator.

These analyses found that, of our three mediators, only involvement with anti-school peers was actually impacted overall by the intervention at two years of follow-up. Intervention impacts on the other two mediator measures did emerge but only at three years of follow-up. Adjustment for the mediators measured at two years did not reduce the size of the intervention effect on bullying victimisation. All this suggested that, at least when looking at all schools together, there was no evidence of mediation by changes in school organisation, student commitment to school or student involvement in anti-school peer groups.[188] In other trials, such mediation analyses have delivered more positive information. In the case of the Welsh exercise referral intervention discussed in the section titled 'Moderation Analyses',[182] mediation analyses suggested that intervention impacts on physical activity were partly explained by increases in participants developing a sense of individual motivation to change their behaviour and by participants benefiting from increasing social support to make these changes.[189] However, on their own, mediation analyses are quite limited from a realist perspective because they do not shed light on how context contributes to the generation of outcomes.

Moderated Mediation Analyses

Moderated mediation analyses assess whether mediation (as explained in the previous section) is contingent on the presence of another factor. They can reveal, for example, that an intervention achieves its effects on a primary outcome via an effect on a certain intermediate outcome but only in some sites or for some individuals. This innovative form of analysis is therefore of obvious value in testing CMOCs because it simultaneously looks at contexts (via moderators), mechanisms (via mediators) and outcomes.

In Learning Together, based on our qualitative findings about mechanisms, we hypothesised that student sense of school belonging would be a key mediator to the intervention reducing bullying victimisation and promoting mental well-being, *but only in some schools*: those that had the opportunity to really major on this aspect of the intervention. To cut a long story short, these analyses suggested that the intervention's effects on reducing bullying victimisation and improving mental well-being were in fact mediated by students' sense of belonging, but that this mediation pathway only occurred in a subgroup of schools with relatively high capacity and low need at baseline. These schools were characterised by good baseline management capacity (as reported by the national school inspectorate), plus already quite high levels of student belonging and already quite low levels of bullying (as reported by students in our baseline survey). In other schools, the intervention was just as effective in reducing bullying and mental distress but these effects appeared not to come about as a result of the intervention increasing student sense of belonging.[190]

Our interpretation of these findings was that in high-capacity/low-stress schools, there was a focus on using the action group to involve students in decision-making and this made students across the school feel more of a sense of belonging in the school community. However, in lower capacity/higher stress schools, schools instead focused on reducing bullying and improving students' mental well-being by using restorative practice to address trouble. In these schools, restorative practice was likely to be a more manageable and immediate way to achieve these benefits, whereas investing in the action group would require more management attention and probably have less immediate impacts. Again, this pathway was also suggested by our qualitative research, reported in the previous chapter. So (at last), our quantitative analyses were starting to shine a light on how the intervention mechanisms might interact with context to generate outcomes. And even better, we were getting broadly the same message from our statistical and qualitative analyses.

In Chapter 4, Section 4.6, we also noted that the healthy context paradox emerged as a potential theory to explain potential intervention harms. While we did not have any qualitative research findings, suggesting this might be a possibility in the case of Learning Together, we did have the data to test whether the healthy context paradox was occurring. We modelled whether the intervention magnified the relationship between bullying victimisation and poor mental health.[191] Our findings suggested that this was not the case.

Qualitative Comparative Analyses

All of the analyses we have so far considered in this chapter rely on probabilistic statistics to look at relatively simple interrelationships. Even the moderated mediation analyses only examine four variables at a time: exposure to the intervention, the moderator, the mediator and the outcome. In reality, mechanisms and how they interact with context to generate outcomes will often be more complex than this. Qualitative comparative analysis (QCA) uses a different approach to examine more complex combinations of conditions that co-occur with an outcome. Rather than using probabilistic statistics, the conditions in question are linked together by the logical connectors 'AND', 'NOT' and 'OR'.[192-194] For example, we might find that the following conditions co-occur with the outcome of a pleasant walk:

nice scenery AND good company NOT (rain OR fog).

Within QCA, a condition is 'necessary' if the outcome cannot occur without the condition being present. A condition is 'sufficient' if the outcome is always present with this condition, regardless of other factors.[195] For example, tea leaves are necessary to make tea. Drinking tea is sufficient to quench thirst. This approach can be applied to understanding what complex combinations of conditions (in our case, contexts and mechanisms) need to be present for an outcome to occur. Qualitative comparative analysis can show not only the combinations of contexts and mechanisms that are necessary or sufficient for an outcome to occur but also those combinations that lead to the outcome *not* occurring.

The first step in any QCA is to build a 'data table' which describes each case, its conditions and outcomes. Table 6.1 shows a hypothetical example of a data table focusing on the example

Table 6.1 Data table for car park prevention of thefts

Case	Indicators of context		Mechanisms		Outcome
Carparks	Police believe a few offenders are responsible for most thefts ('core group context')	Low baseline use of carpark by drivers ('low use context')	CCTV leads to increased rate of arrest and conviction of car thefts (arrest/ removal mechanism)	CCTV leads to increased use of carpark by drivers (natural surveillance mechanism)	Reduction in car thefts
1	1	0	1	0	1
2	0	0	0	0	0
3	1	0	1	0	1
4	1	1	1	1	1
5	0	1	0	1	0
6	0	1	1	0	0
7	1	0	0	1	0
8	0	1	0	1	0

described in Chapter 3 of CCTV in carparks as a means of reducing car thefts. Each row describes a car park with contextual features, mechanisms and outcomes as columns.

The data table suggests that the mechanism of CCTV increasing arrests can generate reduced car thefts but only in the context of a few offenders being responsible for thefts. And the mechanism of increasing natural surveillance can't reduce thefts regardless of context.

After the data table is complete, the focus shifts from cases to the combinations of conditions that lead (or don't lead) to the outcome, which are presented in a 'truth table'.[196] A combination of conditions can be positive (e.g. all car parks within the set report a reduction in thefts), negative (all car parks within the set don't report a reduction in thefts), contradictory (the same combination of conditions produce different results) or residual (possible combinations with no empirical data to test them). For any combination of conditions, one can determine the consistency (in this hypothetical case, the proportion of car parks within each set that have the same outcome) and coverage (i.e. how much of the outcome is explained by the model). When consistency is low, there is weak or contradictory evidence that the combination of conditions co-occurs with the outcome. When coverage is low, this suggests that the model is missing some key explanatory conditions.[196]

The final stage is, where possible, one of Boolean minimisation, which removes any terms which do not add to our explanation of the generation of outcomes. In the case of the car parks, minimisation would leave us with a combination of 'core group context' AND 'arrest/removal mechanism' as the conditions necessary and sufficient for reduction of car thefts. This would account for 100 per cent of the outcomes with 100 per cent consistency in this hypothetical example.

In the Learning Together study, we used QCA to explore how more complex combinations of contextual features and mechanisms appeared to be linked to outcomes.[197] We built our QCA models around the following CMOCs, which differ slightly from those in Chapter 4, Section 4.7, because they reflect what data we had available.

'Sense of belonging' mechanism of benefit: The action group enabled erosion of boundaries between staff and students, and students to increase their sense of belonging in school, making a positive contribution to school, change a broader group of students' attitudes to school and, through this, reductions in bullying. This was particularly important in schools with a pre-existing desire to involve students in decision-making, which enables effective and inclusive action groups.

'Perpetration curtailment' mechanism of benefit: Restorative practice enabled perpetrators to develop a sense of responsibility for their actions and empathy with victims. This generated curtailment of bullying perpetration. This was particularly important in schools where sufficient staff were trained in restorative practice and there were sufficient incidents of bullying to ensure that it was commonly deployed.

'Social and emotional skills' mechanism of benefit: The classroom curriculum and/or the preventative use of restorative practice enabled students to develop social and emotional skills and learn how to resolve conflict, through this, generating reductions in conduct problems and bullying. This was particularly important in schools where students' deficits in social and emotional skills were critical to mechanisms generating bullying.

In testing our hypotheses, we first looked at an overall model in which we assessed whether there was evidence that any or all of these three mechanisms decreased bullying victimisation. This model focused on the mechanisms but not the contexts. We included schools in the intervention and control groups in this analysis because we recognised that these mechanisms could be triggered in some control schools despite their not having access to intervention resources. After this, we drilled down to separately examine whether use of Learning Together resources seemed to trigger each of these three mechanisms and in which contexts, developing a model for each mechanism in turn. These analyses included only schools in the intervention arm since only these had access to the intervention resources. These models focused not on bullying victimisation as an outcome but on the intermediate outcomes that we would expect to be generated by these mechanisms: increased student participation in decisions for the belonging mechanism; decreased bullying perpetration for the perpetration curtailment mechanism; and improved pro-social skills for the social and emotional skills mechanism.

In examining each of these CMOCs, we first constructed a 'data table'. Within the data table, each school formed a case (presented as a row) with contextual features, mechanisms and outcomes as columns. We selected appropriate measures that could serve as proxies for these conditions in our models. In some cases, these drew on quantitative measures used in the student surveys, surveys of action group members or logbooks completed by staff delivering various activities. For example, in the 'social and emotional skills mechanism', we included the following columns: schools where students lacked pro-social skills (contextual feature), drawing on the student baseline questionnaire; schools where students feel unsafe (contextual feature), also drawing on student baselines; schools delivering the social and emotional learning curriculum (potential mechanism), drawing on staff logbooks of delivery; schools using preventative restorative practices (potential mechanism), drawing on staff reports; and improved pro-social behaviour (outcome), based on the follow-up student questionnaire. Because some of the mechanisms that emerged from the qualitative analysis were new, we did not have ready-made quantitative measures of them and so we constructed school-level indicators informed by analysis of qualitative data from each school. For example, we drew on student interviews to develop an indicator of whether in each school restorative practice led to perpetrators developing a sense of empathy. This is common practice within QCAs.

Qualitative comparative analysis can use what are known as 'crisp set' or 'fuzzy set' indicators of conditions. In 'crisp set' QCA, a '1' indicates the presence of a condition or outcome and a '0' indicates its absence. In 'fuzzy set' QCA, the values can range from 0 to 1, indicating their degree of presence of the condition or outcome. We used 'fuzzy set' QCA and therefore had to make judgements for each school as to whether each contextual feature, mechanism and outcome was present, absent or whether this was unclear. For example, in the case of outcomes, we had to assess if there was a significant reduction from baseline to follow-up in that school's rate of bullying. After looking at the data, we judged that schools with greater than 50 per cent reductions were fully cases, schools with less than 15 per cent decreases were definitely not a case and schools with a 30 per cent reduction were unclear. The schools' outcomes were then calibrated, giving every school an indicator score (called a 'truth value') between 0 and 1. A similar process was used for the various markers of each condition. Once this process was completed for every condition, we ran the analysis to get 'truth tables', showing the various possible combinations of conditions and how many schools were within each set. In fuzzy set QCA, data in truth tables are presented as binary, with truth values less than 0.5 being rounded down to 0 and values of 0.5 or more being rounded up to 1.

For the overall model, we found that thirteen schools in the intervention group and thirteen schools in the control group experienced decreased bullying. However, schools in the intervention arm had higher truth values, indicating that they experienced greater decreases in bullying. Moreover, there was more evidence of more hypothesised mechanisms being activated in intervention than control schools. We identified nine combinations of markers of mechanisms that co-occurred with a reduction in bullying. The mechanism with the greatest explanatory power seemed to involve reducing student conduct problems (found in twelve of fifteen effective solutions), which seemed sufficient to reduce bullying regardless of all other factors. This is perhaps not very surprising and doesn't tell us anything about how reductions in conduct problems came about. Other combinations of conditions also were linked to reductions in bullying. For example, some schools seemed to reduce bullying by teaching students social and emotional skills and how to resolve conflict despite not achieving improvements in student belonging or curtailing perpetration through restorative practice. But these analyses shed limited light on mechanisms because they don't consider how they were triggered by the intervention or how they interacted with context to generate outcomes.

Next, we drilled down to examine each of the three mechanisms described earlier in this section, and how the use of Learning Together resources seemed to trigger these to generate intermediate outcomes and in which contexts. These analyses included only schools in the intervention arm since only these had access to the intervention resources. In terms of our three mechanisms, we found evidence that student participation in decisions was improved when students felt they had made a positive contribution to the action group and action group members felt that they were successful in initiating broader change in student attitudes to their school. Bullying perpetration was reduced in schools having sufficient staff trained in restorative practice. Student pro-social skills were improved when schools delivered preventative restorative practice (but schools did not need to deliver the social and emotional skills curriculum) and in schools where more students felt unsafe at baseline. Our hypothesised contextual conditions were important in fewer models than we had expected but they still exerted influence in some. We found little evidence, for example, that restorative practice needed high baseline levels of bullying at a school for the de-escalation mechanism to operate, or that schools needed to have students with deficits in social and emotional skills for the social and emotional skills mechanism to work. There was also some evidence that schools with more baseline need had to activate more mechanisms to achieve the same benefit as schools with fewer problems. Qualitative comparative analysis thus enabled us to explore generative explanations in terms of complex combinations of contextual features and mechanisms, suggesting there were multiple pathways to the same outcome.[198] Our research also suggested that, while a single mechanism could be sufficient to decrease bullying in some schools, multiple mechanisms have to be activated together to reduce bullying in other schools.[199]

Box 6.1 Summary of refinement of Learning Together CMOCs informed by quantitative research conducted in the outcome evaluation

'Sense of Belonging' Mechanism of Benefit

Context: Particularly in schools with strong organisational capacity and an inclusive culture which enables effective and inclusive action groups, and particularly for boys and those experiencing bullying at baseline but with no differences by socio-economic status.

Mechanism: The action group enables reclassification and reframing in schools, so that boundaries between staff and students are eroded, students feel they have made a positive contribution to the school and mutual empathy is engendered.

Outcome: Generating increased student sense of belonging in school, increased commitment to school pro-social norms and reduced bullying and aggression.

'Perpetration Curtailment' Mechanism of Benefit

Context: Particularly in schools where a critical mass of staff commit to delivering restorative practice but with no differences according to baseline level of bullying.

Mechanism: Restorative practice enables perpetrators to develop responsibility for actions and empathy with victims.

Outcome: Generating curtailment of bullying perpetration and aggression.

'Social and Emotional Skills' Mechanism of Benefit

Context: Particularly in schools where staff commit to delivering restorative practice but with no difference according to levels of baseline social and emotional skills.

Mechanism: The preventative use of restorative practice (much more than the social and emotional skills curriculum) enabled students to develop social and emotional skills.

Outcome: Generating avoidance of conflict and reductions in bullying and aggression level.

6.3 Drawing on Multiple Analyses to Refine Context–Mechanism–Outcome Configurations

In Box 6.1, we summarise how we came to see our CMOCs after testing them through various quantitative analyses.

This chapter has explored how CMOCs may be tested using quantitative data from 'phase III' trials examining intervention effectiveness. We have seen how analyses of overall outcomes, moderation, mediation and moderated mediation, as well as QCA, can offer nuanced insights into how intervention mechanisms might generate outcomes and on what contextual factors this is contingent.

Our analyses of the overall outcomes of Learning Together provide no indication of mechanisms or contexts but are nonetheless still useful, especially for public health interventions where the focus is often on population-level effects. Mediator analyses start to offer insights into mechanisms but not how these interact with context. Moderator analyses examine how effects might vary with context (in terms of place and person) but don't tell us much about how the mechanisms actually operate. Conducted separately, such analyses still do not allow direct testing of CMOCs. Moderated mediation analyses put the two together so that, for the first time, we can start to test hypotheses about how mechanisms generate impacts in interaction with context. While powerful, the limitation of this form of analysis is that it can only examine what are still relatively simple combinations of contexts and mechanisms.

Qualitative comparative analysis offers a means to look at more elaborate combinations of contextual features and mechanisms, and how these co-occur with detected outcomes. However, a disadvantage of such analyses is that because they do not involve probabilistic statistics, they may be undermined by chance co-occurrences in which coincidences are misinterpreted as indicating causality. Small sample sizes make this more likely. They also often draw on crude markers of conditions or outcomes. For example, our measure of bullying reduction represented the trend over time within a school with no control of other factors influencing this. Our measure of whether restorative practice enabling perpetrators to develop empathy drew only on qualitative data.

We saw that QCA can draw on information from both arms in a randomised trial (or, indeed, a quasi-experimental study with a non-randomised control group). Such analyses can shed light on how mechanisms interact with context to generate outcomes in either arm, and whether there is more evidence for such generation of outcomes in the intervention compared to the control group. An advantage of drawing on randomised trials to provide the data for QCA is that comparisons between arms are balanced and fair. Qualitative comparative analyses cannot adjust for baseline differences because they do not use probabilistic statistics. As a result, QCA making comparisons between the arms of quasi-experimental studies are less likely to involve balanced and fair comparisons because of baseline differences between arms.

These CMOCs offer nuanced information about how the Learning Together intervention works, where and for whom. It does so based on rigorous evidence. It should provide much more useful evidence to policymakers and school staff considering whether to use Learning Together or similar approaches elsewhere. Most importantly, it suggests that schools may need to take different approaches to preventing bullying depending on their baseline capacity and ethos. Schools with strong capacity and relatively low levels of challenge may opt to implement all aspects of the whole-school change intervention.

Schools with less management capacity and facing more challenges at baseline may choose to address bullying incrementally, starting with the (relatively) easy step of training staff to use restorative practice. Our analyses should also provide academic researchers with information about how school environments can influence student health, and about the validity of the theory of human functioning and school organisation in explaining this. We return to these questions of the use of evidence in policy and academia in chapters 9 and 10.

In the preceding two chapters, we have considered the value and means of conducting realist evaluations within single trials or other outcome evaluation studies. Single studies (randomised or otherwise) will always be limited in what light they can shed on how intervention mechanisms interact with context to generate outcomes. This is because any one study will be located in a particular region or country and therefore will only encompass a fairly limited diversity of settings and populations. If properly conducted and able to include sufficient studies providing the information needed, systematic reviews should be able to shed much more light on CMOCs because they should be able to draw on a wider diversity of context. However, as we saw in chapters 2 and 3, systematic reviews currently provide very limited insights into what works for whom and how. Realist reviews, while focused on much more apt questions, are less useful than they could be because of the methodological limitations described in Chapter 3. In the next chapter, we therefore examine how systematic reviews might be reoriented towards examining more useful questions while retaining their undoubted methodological strengths. We call this approach realist systematic review.

Building and Refining Realist Theory in Systematic Reviews

7.1 The Current Limitations of Systematic Reviews and Realist Reviews

As we saw in Chapter 3, systematic reviews focusing on questions about 'what works' still rarely examine how, in what context and for whom interventions work.[67 200] These evidence reviews typically only focus on determining the overall effects associated with interventions, informing whether public health interventions can be accredited as 'effective' or not. They do not test hypotheses about how intervention mechanisms interact with context to generate outcomes. Meta-analyses tend to focus on aggregating included studies to determine overall effect sizes, often neglecting to examine whether intervention studies report different effect estimates in different contexts, or what mediators account for such effects. This means that it is usually impossible for those reading a systematic review to get a clear sense of how an intervention works, or in which populations and settings it will work best. This is clearly the case, for example, in previous systematic reviews of the effects of youth development interventions, which have been shown to be simultaneously effective, ineffective and harmful in different studies with little explanation of why this might be.[201-203]

This approach is associated with the increasing popularity of clearing houses for effective interventions, such as the US *Blueprints Youth Programmes* resource (www.blueprintspro grams.com/) and the UK *Investing in Children* database (http://investinginchildren.eu/). These list 'effective' interventions without considering in which settings and for which populations they might be appropriate. Although a few systematic reviews do examine how the effects of interventions vary by demographic subgroup or setting of implementation,[71 73] systematic reviews rarely examine what might explain any heterogeneity found in intervention effects. This is partly because included studies rarely report on these factors in a consistent way.[204]

We saw in Chapter 3 that realist reviews have been proposed as an alternative method for synthesising evidence that is attentive to context and mechanism. However, we argued that realist reviews are insufficiently led by protocols, insufficiently comprehensive in their searches, insufficiently attentive to study quality and insufficiently rigorous in how they synthesise evidence. They generally limit synthesis to exploring whether the narratives of results reported in included studies align with the review CMOCs rather than critically appraising and synthesising the evidence presented in included studies to test CMOCs. In this and the next chapter, we describe a method for systematic reviews which aims to broaden their scope so that they can consider questions of context and mechanism while retaining the use of protocols and safeguarding the rigour with which the reviews search for, assess the quality of and synthesise evidence. We call this approach 'realist systematic reviews'. Such reviews can continue to synthesise evidence of overall effects (including via meta-analysis where appropriate) while also undertaking other syntheses drawing on broader forms of evidence to better understand how interventions work, for whom they are beneficial or harmful and how this might vary with context.

7.2 Our Case Study: A Systematic Review of School-based Interventions to Prevention Dating/Relationship Violence and/or Gender Violence

In this and the next chapter, we use our own systematic review of school-based interventions to prevent dating and relationship violence (DRV) and/or gender-based violence (GBV) among young people as a case study to show how we go about conducting realist thinking and analyses within a systematic review. In this chapter, we will focus on how systematic reviews can synthesise intervention descriptions, theories of change and process evaluations of included studies to build and refine intervention theories of change and CMOCs. This parallels the use of qualitative research to develop and refine CMOCs in randomised trials.

We were motivated to undertake our review because we observed that conventional systematic reviews have not been very useful in informing policy about DRV and GBV prevention among young people. This is concerning because DRV and GBV are serious problems which are common among adolescents all over the world and which cause significant harms.[205] [206] Existing systematic reviews offer little guidance for developing and delivering prevention interventions. For example, one systematic review pooled intervention effects on DRV from multiple studies, finding no overall evidence of effectiveness but plenty of heterogeneity in effects between studies, which was not explained.[207] The review did not examine questions of implementation or causal mechanisms. Other systematic reviews focused on DRV and GBV prevention among young people have also not addressed these questions.[208-211]

In the systematic review we report here, we defined DRV as physical, sexual and emotional violence within relationships between young people. We defined GBV as violence rooted in gender/sexual inequality outside dating relationships. We included randomised trials and process evaluations of school-based interventions aiming to prevent DRV and/or GBV in terms of victimisation and/or perpetration among students aged five to eighteen years. We included randomised trials and not non-randomised studies because we knew that it was feasible and appropriate for schools to be randomly allocated to deliver DRV/GBV interventions. We also included mediation and moderation analyses reported in papers linked to relevant randomised trials (also known as 'trial sibling evidence'). The review searched twenty-one databases and used a variety of other methods to identify relevant studies. All these searches identified over 40,000 unique references, out of which we identified 68 trials and 137 process evaluations based on a review of titles, abstracts and then full studies where necessary.

Synthesising Intervention Descriptions to Categorise Interventions and 'Track' Intended Mechanisms

Using the terminology employed in realist reviews, the first task is to 'track' CMOCs: in other words, to define a theory of change for the intervention and use this to develop and refine CMOCs. In the case of our review, to start this process of tracking, we first aimed to examine studies' descriptions of interventions and to use this to categorise the interventions based on their aims and components, and start to understand their intended mechanisms. We did this 'inductively' using the descriptions of interventions to build up a taxonomy that allowed us to place each intervention into a discrete category.

We found that most interventions aimed to equip young people with the personal capabilities and motivations needed for them to prevent DRV/GBV. For example, interventions such as 'DAT-E Adolescence' aimed to stop DRV or GBV by helping students understand the unacceptability of these behaviours. We put such interventions into a 'basic safety' mechanism category.[212]

Other interventions, such as the 'DRV Curriculum' intervention, aimed not only to stop negative behaviours, such as perpetration and victimisation, but also to promote positive behaviours such as conflict management or healthy relationship behaviours. We put these interventions into a 'positive development' mechanism category.[213]

Interventions in both these categories included similar student components such as the guided practising of skills; group discussions; individual reflection; visual/image- or narrative-based learning; or student competitions in class. Both categories also included staff components such as training.

A few interventions, such as the 'Good Schools Toolkit', had even broader aims, to modify the social or physical environment in schools as a way to prevent DRV/GBV. We put such interventions into a 'school transformation' mechanism category.[214] Such interventions included components such as changes to school policies, participative planning of activities, school clubs, displaying visual materials in shared space and monitoring the safety of school spaces.

Synthesising Intervention Theories of Change to Further 'Track' Intended Mechanisms

The next task is to synthesise intervention theories of change as they are described in included process and outcome evaluations. We recommend using meta-ethnographic methods to do this.[215] Meta-ethnography is a method that was first developed to synthesise findings from multiple qualitative studies. It uses quite similar methods to those used within a single qualitative study to analyse findings from multiple interviews or focus group discussions. As we described in Chapter 5, qualitative analysis often proceeds via three key steps. Firstly, it identifies recurring themes, whereby different people express similar experiences or ideas but using different language. Secondly, qualitative analysis involves looking for cases where the ideas expressed in different interviews seem to contradict each other. The researcher then refines the analysis so that it can explain such differences. Thirdly, qualitative analysis often builds up an overall picture of some social phenomenon by piecing together the partial views of this phenomenon expressed in different interviews or focus groups.

Meta-ethnography was designed to use these three processes but applied to developing an analysis across multiple primary qualitative studies rather than multiple interviews or focus groups. Within meta-ethnography, these processes are referred to as reciprocal translation (the same concepts described in different terms between studies); refutational synthesis (contradictions in the concepts expressed in different studies); and line of argument (where the concepts from different studies allow us to build a bigger picture than is available in any one study).[215] Our synthesis started off by applying these meta-ethnographic approaches, not to qualitative studies but instead to the descriptions of theories of change in different studies.

We wanted to see whether they expressed common concepts, whether they differed from each other in important ways and whether they could be drawn together to build up a more comprehensive theory of change for school-based prevention of DRV/GBV.

In our review, we aimed to identify an overall theory of change for this type of intervention as well as develop theories of change for each category of intervention.[216] Our meta-ethnography of intervention theories of change was also informed by the theory of human functioning and school organisation (the same theory that underpinned Learning Together) and the Capability–Opportunity–Motivation Behaviour (COM-B) framework to help us make sense of and synthesise these theories. We felt that both of these theories provided a useful way of understanding how schools might promote changes in behaviour, which we believed strongly resonated with our reading of the theories of change that we found in our studies. We have already described the theory of human functioning and school organisation in Chapter 4. The COM-B framework proposes that behaviour is enabled when people possess the capability (e.g. the knowledge and skills), opportunity (e.g. the autonomy and resources) and motivation (e.g. the intention or attitudes) to implement that behaviour.[144] We used these theories as a 'lens' to sensitise us to the key concepts and therefore aid our interpretation of the theories of change we came across. This is perfectly normal in meta-ethnography, as it is when analysing qualitative data from interviews or focus group discussions.[93]

Using these methods, we further developed our understanding of how interventions might work.[216] We identified that both the 'basic safety' and 'positive development' mechanisms aim to build individual or group motivations or capabilities that help prevent initiation or escalation of DRV/GBV. The 'basic safety' mechanism aims to shut down negative behaviours by modifying motivations, for example, by making clear that DRV and GBV are unacceptable. The 'positive development' mechanism goes beyond this to promoting positive behaviours, for example, aiming to develop young people's skills in managing conflict or building healthy relationships.

The 'school transformation' mechanism aims to transform how schools are organised to promote students' sense of belonging and acceptance of pro-social norms. We theorised that the school transformation mechanism involved 'de-classification'. As we explained in Chapter 5, this is defined in the theory of human functioning and school organisation as eroding 'boundaries' (i.e. strengthening relationships) between staff and students, academic and broader personal development and schools and local communities. It could also involve eroding boundaries between the classroom and wider school, and different professional roles within the school. However, in an example of refutational synthesis, we saw that some interventions delivered in high crime areas involved a mechanism that actually built up boundaries between the school and the local community to reject pro-violence community norms. The school transformation mechanism also involved 'reframing', defined in the theory of human functioning and school organisation as increasing student participation in decisions in the classroom and wider school so that schooling is re-centred on student needs and preferences. We theorised that 'de-classification' and 'reframing' in turn increase student belonging and acceptance of pro-social norms leading to reduced DRV and GBV. We then drew on these synthesised theories of change to 'track' the mechanism element of CMOCs.

We hypothesised that the 'basic safety' mechanism is triggered by school staff using intervention resources to enact relatively simple interventions, such as school lessons on preventing DRV and/or GBV. Student involvement in such lessons motivates them to prevent DRV and GBV by encouraging them to develop more negative attitudes to these forms of violence. These lessons also enable students to develop the very basic level of knowledge and skills which provide them with the capability needed to avoid it. In turn, these enable students to avoid and/or challenge DRV and/or GBV.

We hypothesised that the 'positive development' mechanism is triggered by school staff using intervention resources to enact slightly more complex interventions involving single or multiple components. These operate in classrooms, extracurricular activities, school discipline systems or some other single level of school organisation. Student involvement in these activities encourages them to develop a set of capabilities and motivations that go beyond merely the avoidance of violence to include, for example, conflict negotiation or maintaining healthy relationships. In turn, these enable students to be less involved in DRV and/or GBV.

We hypothesised that the school transformation mechanism is triggered by school staff using intervention resources to enact much more complex interventions involving multiple components operating at multiple levels of school organisation. These transform schools via reclassification (eroding boundaries between staff and students, the classroom and wider school, schools and local communities and different professional roles within the school) and reframing (schooling centred on student needs and preferences). Student involvement in these transformed school structures encourages them to develop a greater sense of belonging at school and increased acceptance of school social norms. In turn, this motivates students to be less involved in DRV and/or GBV behaviour.

We hypothesised that the 'basic safety' and 'positive development' mechanisms would generate smaller reductions in DRV and GBV because they operate at fewer different levels of school organisation. We also thought that these mechanisms would be less sustainable because they do not result in enduring changes in school structures and require constant re-implementation to renew any impacts. We hypothesised that the school transformation mechanism would generate larger effects and be more sustainable because it affected different levels of school organisations and aimed to bring about enduring changes to these. Our synthesis of intervention theories of change did not offer many insights into how these three mechanisms might interact with different contexts to generate different outcomes because the theories did not consider contexts. To further 'track' our CMOCs so that these considered context, we turned to synthesising the process evaluations.

Synthesising Process Evaluations to Refine to Better Understand the Importance of Context

It is also useful to draw on process evaluations to refine our understandings of how intervention mechanisms might interact with context to generate outcomes. This is analogous to the use of qualitative research within trials. It is especially useful in systematic reviews because it sheds light on the potential importance of context, something that intervention theories of change will often lack much consideration of, as we saw in Chapter 4.[109] [110] Synthesis of process evaluation can deepen our understanding of how contextual features, in terms of providers, settings and recipients, might influence implementation and receipt, which can shed light on how mechanisms might be theorised to interact with context. Again, meta-ethnographic methods can be used, aiming to identify cases of reciprocal translation, refutational synthesis and line of argument synthesis across the process evaluations included in the review.

In the case of our review, we first assessed the quality of the process evaluations using the 'EPPI-Centre' tool.[217] This assesses the process evaluations in terms of whether their sampling encompasses a diversity of experiences and views, whether study findings are informed by data, whether the study prioritises the perspectives of participants and how broad and deep their findings are.

Our synthesis of process evaluation identified that implementation was facilitated by schools having adequate resources and leadership to support this, and by schools being committed to preventing DRV and GBV. It was hindered by schools experiencing time constraints and competing priorities. These findings were consistent with other syntheses of evidence on the implementation of health-focused interventions in schools.[136] [218] [219] Interventions were also better implemented if they were easier for staff to deliver and could be adapted to suit a particular school. These last findings suggested how we might refine our CMOCs to account for context.

Box 7.1 CMOCs for school-based prevention of DRV/GBV informed by synthesis of intervention descriptions, theories of change and process evaluations

'Basic Safety' Mechanism of Benefit

Context: Particularly in schools which lack the time, resources, leadership and commitment to deliver more difficult interventions.

Mechanism: School staff deliver simple activities aiming to prevent or stop DRV and GBV by making clear that DRV and GBV are unacceptable.

Outcome: Generating small and unsustained reductions in DRV and GBV by promoting the motivations and capabilities needed to do this.

'Positive Development' Mechanism of Benefit

Context: Particularly in schools which lack the time, resources, leadership and commitment to deliver more difficult interventions.

Mechanism: School staff enact interventions involving single or multiple components aiming to develop students' positive development.

Outcome: Generating small and unsustained reductions in DRV and GBV but students developing capabilities and motivations going beyond merely the avoidance of violence to include, for example, conflict negotiation or maintaining healthy relationships.

'School Transformation' Mechanism of Benefit

Context: Particularly in schools which have the time, resources, leadership and commitment to deliver more difficult interventions.

Mechanism: Schools are transformed via erosion of boundaries (between staff and students, the classroom and wider school, schools and local communities and different professional roles within the school) and reframing (schooling centred on student needs and preferences).

Outcome: Generating large and sustained increases in students' sense of belonging and acceptance of school social norms and through this reduced DRV and GBV.

We hypothesised that the 'basic safety' and 'positive development' mechanisms would be most likely to generate reductions in DRV and GBV in schools which lacked the time, resources, leadership and commitment to deliver more complex, difficult interventions. Such schools would struggle to deliver interventions aiming to trigger the 'school transformation' mechanism. We hypothesised that the 'school transformation' mechanism would nonetheless generate the largest and most sustained reductions in DRV and GBV but only in schools with the time, resources, leadership and commitment to support this. These are summarised in Box 7.1.

In this chapter, we have explored how systematic reviews can be broadened in scope to examine questions not only of what works but also how interventions work, where and for whom. The chapter has focused on how such reviews can 'track' theory: developing a theory of change and CMOCs for the intervention type being reviewed, based on syntheses of reported intervention descriptions, theories of change and process evaluations. In the next chapter, we explore how reviews can test these theories of change and CMOCs.

Chapter

8

Testing Realist Theory through Synthesising Outcome Evaluations

In Chapters 2 and 7, we discussed how most systematic reviews synthesise evidence on intervention effects to answer questions about 'what works'. They tend not to examine broader evidence to understand questions of implementation, mechanisms or context.[67 201] In Chapter 7, we described how systematic reviews can be broadened in scope to understand intervention theories of change, explore evidence on how context influences implementation and draw on this to 'track' CMOCs.

8.1 How Our Approach to Analysis Differs from Conventional Systematic Reviews and Realist Reviews

In this chapter, we examine how systematic reviews can synthesise quantitative evidence in innovative ways to test, augment and refine these CMOCs. As we described in Chapter 2, the analysis of quantitative data in most systematic reviews does not attend much to context. It tends to pool the effect sizes reported from included studies, appearing to assume that there will be a single underlying true effect across studies which pooling will reveal.[44] This would be useful if interventions really did work the same way across settings and populations, which might be true of some biomedical interventions and perhaps a few complex social interventions, but it is not useful where effects vary for good reason across contexts. Some systematic reviews do report on subgroup effects either according to characteristics of setting or population,[71 73] and this can help inform us about interventions' potential for transfer to other settings and populations. However, without a fuller theorisation of how interventions work and how they interact with context, such insights will be quite limited.[55] In this chapter, we examine what innovative quantitative analyses can be done within systematic reviews to test, augment and refine CMOCs, and thereby develop a better understanding of how interventions work and in which contexts they will work best.

The approach we describe is very different from that used in traditional realist reviews. We saw in Chapter 3 that these aim to test and refine their CMOCs by seeing how the CMOCs align with the narratives presented by included studies. Such reviews aim to include a purposive sample of studies offering diverse perspectives not limited to a specific study design. Such reviews aim to judge the validity of specific findings and not the overall quality of methods. In contrast, we believe that the outcome evaluations synthesised need to use designs that are rigorous and appropriate for the intervention in question. We believe that we need to assess the quality of included studies to inform what weight we give their results. This should ensure that reviews offer the most rigorous means of examining the CMOCs. We believe that the included studies must be a comprehensive set of all such studies out there, rather than merely being a purposive set of studies offering diverse perspectives.

And we believe that examining CMOCs instead requires reviewers to examine whether the empirical regularities (and not merely the narratives) reported in empirical outcome evaluations are in line with what our 'tracked' CMOCs would predict.

8.2 Overview of the Quantitative Analyses We Used in Our Review of Prevention of Dating and Relationship Violence, and Gender-Based Violence

The analyses we recommend to use within realist systematic reviews include meta-analyses examining an intervention's overall effects but also network meta-analyses examining the effectiveness of different intervention components, analyses examining how intervention effects differ between settings and populations and what mediators seem to be important.[220-224] As with Chapter 7, we use the example of our systematic review of school-based interventions to prevent DRV and GBV.[225] The outcome evaluations that we included in this review were required to use the randomised controlled trial design. We made this decision based on the fact that the interventions we had in mind could feasibly be evaluated using this least biased of outcome evaluation designs. We knew that such studies had been conducted and that schools were prepared to join studies knowing they had a chance of either being allocated to receive the intervention or be in the control group. So, in this case, we decided we did not need to include other studies which would likely offer more biased estimates of effect because they did not involve such fair comparisons. However, in the case of systematic reviews of other sorts of interventions, it would be appropriate to admit other designs when it was felt that inclusion of only randomised trials would not allow inclusion of sufficient evidence because of the challenges in random allocation, use of control groups and/or use of prospective data.[172] We reported in the previous chapter that in the case of our review of DRV and GBV prevention interventions, our searches identified sixty-eight trials, which form the basis of the analyses reported here. We used narrative synthesis and statistical meta-analysis, as well as network meta-analyses, harvest plots, meta-regression and qualitative comparative analysis (QCA) to analyse these studies.

Meta-analysis to Assess Overall Effects

It is right to be sceptical about whether overall meta-analyses will reveal an overall intervention effect for a particular intervention approach that would homogeneously apply across populations and settings. Nonetheless, these are still worth conducting as a starting point. Such analyses might still give some sense of the overall population health potential of an intervention approach: whether the mechanism that is triggered by the interventions appears to generate outcomes across settings or not. And they can also provide a starting point and point of comparison for other, more nuanced analyses.

In the case of our review, we found that there was an overall effect of school-based prevention on DRV perpetration and victimisation in the long term (one year or longer post-baseline) but not in the short term.[225] We interpreted that this may be because interventions require at least one year to bed down in schools and impact on dating relationships. Interventions aiming to trigger 'school transformation' mechanisms in particular would take time to modify the school environment. Even those interventions aiming to trigger basic safety or positive development mechanisms would likely take time to reduce DRV because impacts might only manifest once students begin dating or embark on new relationships in which they had the opportunity to apply new capabilities or motivations.[226]

Our meta-analyses found no overall intervention impacts on GBV victimisation or perpetration. We interpreted that this might reflect the fact that, whereas DRV tends to be a behaviour enacted in private within dating and relationships, GBV is often a more public activity, such as sexual harassment.[227] As a result, DRV might be more amenable to change when young people in relationships learn how to avoid this, whereas GBV might be more influenced by collective peer social norms, which are harder to modify.

Network Meta-analysis to Explore Variations in Outcomes by Intervention Components

A technique called network meta-analysis can also be useful to examine whether differences in the combinations of intervention components might account for differences in reported effects between studies. Network meta-analyses allow comparison of effectiveness between pairs of interventions. In normal meta-analyses, such pair-wise comparisons require that included studies actually report empirical comparisons between different intervention groups. Network meta-analyses allow such comparisons even when there are no empirical studies, including these direct comparisons. They do this by drawing on a network of included studies which might, for example, compare each of a pair of interventions to a similar comparator even if not to each other, thus allowing an indirect comparison between the pair.[228]

Our use of this approach in our review involved grouping interventions in ways that were suggested by our tracking of CMOCs, classifying interventions in terms of their components and which levels of school organisation they addressed.[225] This analysis did not provide very clear evidence of certain components being more effective than others. However, there was some suggestion that simple, single-component interventions were (contrary to our tracked CMOC hypotheses) more effective than more complex interventions in preventing long-term DRV victimisation and perpetration. We interpreted that this might be because these simpler interventions are more feasible to deliver in more schools. Even if the mechanism that these simple interventions trigger might have less potential for generating reductions in DRV, the fact that these interventions are easier to deliver might mean that their impacts mount up more over time. Or it might be that these simpler interventions allow a narrower but more intense focus on preventing DRV.

Reviewing Mediation Analyses to Understand Mechanisms

In Chapter 6, we discussed the use of mediation analysis within trials to shed light on intervention mechanism. These can also be used in realist systematic reviews to start to understand how the mechanisms triggered by interventions might generate outcomes, although they offer no insights into how such mechanisms interact with context to do this. There is no means of statistically pooling mediation analyses from primary studies so these are just narratively synthesised (described). However, unlike in a realist review, this narrative synthesis involves the reviewer examining statistical reports from included studies and writing a narrative summarising these. In contrast, a realist review qualitatively synthesises the narratives reported in included studies, hopefully checking these against the reported statistics to ensure they are accurate.

An important point to note is that the analyses that we can do in a systematic review are much less within our control than is the case for the analyses we do within a trial or other primary study. For example, in a trial we can ensure that we collect data on the potential mediators we are interested in, to ensure that we can test our CMOCs. However, in a systematic review we do not have this control. The extent to which we can examine mediation or moderation is determined by what variables studies include, and what analyses they run and report. This will be apparent in the analyses we discuss in the rest of this chapter. We cannot always ensure that our analyses of mediation or moderation align perfectly with the CMOCs that we wish to test. Instead, we have to take a more inductive approach, summarising the evidence reported by primary studies and then reflecting what, if anything, it tells us about our CMOCs and how these might be refined or augmented.

In the case of our review, we found that there was some evidence from mediation analyses that, where interventions were effective in preventing DRV victimisation and perpetration, this was mediated by them causing students to be more likely to see such violence as unacceptable. There was also patchy evidence from some, but not all, studies that interventions might work by enabling students to become more knowledgeable about DRV. There was no evidence that conflict management skills, bystander actions or student sense of school belonging were mediators. Our interpretation was that these analyses added to the picture that school-based interventions primarily reduce DRV via a mechanism involving the building of individual capabilities and motivations, particularly in terms of creating more negative attitudes towards violence in order to increase motivation to prevent this.

Turning from DRV to GBV, there was evidence from only one study that improved student sense of school belonging was a mediator of intervention effects on reduced GBV victimisation and perpetration.[229] We interpreted this evidence, despite its paucity, as supporting the view that, where interventions were successful in reducing GBV, this was most likely to occur via a school transformation mechanism. However, the analyses suggested that interventions did not generally achieve this impact and the mediation analyses did not tell us in which schools the mechanism was most likely to be effective. In addition, there is a broader issue that mediation analyses are only conducted when interventions are effective; they suggest why effective interventions are effective, but do not tell us why ineffective interventions are ineffective. This leads onto our next analyses, which focused on questions of context and moderation.

Reviewing Moderation Analyses to Understand Variation in Outcomes by Context

Within realist systematic reviews, moderation analyses, as is the case within trials, can be used to assess whether interventions increase or decrease health inequalities, and to start to understand how intervention mechanisms might interact with context to generate different outcomes in different settings or with different populations. Our syntheses of moderation evidence within our review were also mostly narrative. As was the case with evidence on mediation, we could not control what moderators were examined in included studies and could only synthesise what evidence was available and then reflect what it might tell us about how we need to augment or modify our CMOCs. In this sense, our analyses of moderation were largely inductive rather than hypothesis-testing. Narrative syntheses of moderation analyses reported by included studies suggested that intervention effects on DRV victimisation did not differ by students' gender, age, ethnicity, sexual orientation, dating history, prior experience of DRV victimisation or acculturation.

Turning from DRV victimisation to perpetration, our narrative synthesis of moderation analyses reported in studies found that multiple studies reported evidence that intervention effects were greater for boys' perpetration and some studies reported evidence that effects were greater for those who had previously perpetrated DRV. Our interpretation of this was that these interventions may have been interpreted by students as focusing primarily on preventing male perpetration. Informed by the above findings on mediation, these interventions might have achieved these effects by changing boys' attitudes to violence, perhaps particularly among those who had previously been perpetrators. While these findings about subgroup effects are useful, they are hypothesis-generating rather than conclusive, because subgroup analyses are especially susceptible to reporting bias (e.g. not publishing 'uninteresting' subgroup analyses) or substandard reporting (e.g. just reporting findings as 'not significant', which was a problem in our systematic review).

Meta-regression to Explore Variation in Outcomes by Context

Meta-regression refers to analyses conducted within systematic reviews which assess the association of multiple study-level variables with differences in effect estimates reported by different studies.[230] Such analyses require that enough studies all report on the same variables so that an analysis can identify statistically significant patterns. Although it is the reviewer who runs the meta-regression, and therefore has more control over what moderators are examined, this control is still highly limited. Only study-level variables, such as the proportion of the sample who are female or the sample's average age, rather than within-study variables, such as each participant's gender or age, can be assessed. And the reviewer can only examine variables which all studies included in the analyses report. Furthermore, meta-regression analyses are, at best, hypothesis-building or refining, rather than conclusive. Because they focus on study-level descriptors, interpretation of their results can be subject to the ecological fallacy, where differences between groups (such as the proportion of a trial sample who are female) are assumed to indicate differences within groups (whether individual participants are female).[231]

In our review, we were able to run some meta-regressions to further examine moderation. These did not align closely with our CMOCs and were instead mainly inductive in orientation. There was some evidence from the meta-regressions which we ran that interventions achieved bigger reductions in DRV victimisation in schools where girls formed a larger proportion of those involved in intervention activities. We interpreted this as evidence that school interventions might be more effective where a critical mass of girls encouraged greater student engagement and the de-normalisation of male violence. We did not take it as evidence that interventions achieve bigger reductions in DRV victimisation for individual girls than individual boys as this would have been an example of the ecological fallacy.

There was also evidence of long-term reductions of GBV victimisation and perpetration reported from studies in high- but not low-income countries. We interpreted that this might be because GBV could be reduced by longer term school transformations or other intervention mechanisms that could only be triggered in schools with higher capacity, with these being more likely to be present in high-income countries. Intervention components were another possible factor. We also used meta-regression to test whether there were any differences in effect according to the components that made up interventions, but found no evidence for this.

Qualitative Comparative Analysis to Understand What Combinations of Factors Were Linked to Outcomes

In Chapter 6, we described how QCA can be used to understand what combinations of markers of contexts and mechanisms co-occur with outcomes. We applied this to exploring what combinations of markers of mechanisms and school contexts were linked to reductions in bullying victimisation within our trial of Learning Together. Qualitative comparative analysis can also be used to see patterns of impact within systematic reviews.[232] Each intervention-control comparison reported in an included study forms a case (and a row in the data table). Columns then indicate what conditions are present for each case.[195] A truth table then identifies what different combinations of conditions are represented by studies and the extent to which these co-occur with an outcome.[196][233] As is the case with the other analyses that we apply to realist systematic reviews, we have to base what our QCAs examine on what information is reported by included studies. We therefore have less power to focus our QCAs precisely on the CMOCs that we wish to test. In this sense, the QCAs we apply within a realist systematic review are more inductive than those we would conduct within a primary evaluation. All we can do is run the QCAs that are possible and then reflect on what they might tell us about how to refine our CMOCs.

Other than for short-term DRV perpetration (where no patterns were apparent), our QCAs were able to identify a set of conditions that provided pathways towards the greatest impact. We found that a key condition for reduced victimisation was reduced perpetration, which applied across short-term and long-term DRV victimisation and short-term GBV perpetration. While not surprising, the fact that this result has obvious face validity increased our confidence that these QCAs were providing valid results. Several other pathways towards reduction of victimisation were apparent: for example, interventions including a single-gender component or targeting a population with a critical mass of girls. It was important that interventions targeted a critical mass of girls for interventions which went beyond a single component.

We also found some evidence that certain intervention components were actually a barrier to impacts. For long-term DRV victimisation, parental involvement was one such 'effect depleting' component. For short-term GBV victimisation, victims of GBV coming to a school to tell their story was another such effect depleting component. Our interpretation was that these intervention components could inadvertently lead to students receiving conflicting messages from those they received from teachers about the nature of GBV and how it could be prevented.

Qualitative comparative analysis suggested that, to prevent long-term DRV perpetration and short-term GBV perpetration, the most effective intervention components provided opportunities for guided practice of skills and attitudes, and focused on student relationships. These analyses also suggested that, to prevent short-term GBV (but not DRV) perpetration, the most effective interventions involved components aiming to transform school social environments.

8.3 Drawing on These Analyses to Refine Context–Mechanism–Outcome Configurations

We refined our CMOCs in the light of these analyses. We concluded that school-based interventions can be effective in triggering mechanisms to reduce DRV perpetration and, through this, victimisation in the long but not the short term. However, these interventions are not generally effective in triggering mechanisms that can prevent GBV victimisation or perpetration. These outcomes take time to be generated because of the time taken for individuals to apply the capabilities and motivations learnt in relationships.

These interventions generally work not by transforming school environments or promoting positive development but via a basic safety mechanism focusing on encouraging students to develop capabilities and motivation concerning the unacceptability of violence. This mechanism particularly reduces DRV perpetration among males and those with previous experience of perpetration, and when delivered to school populations with a critical mass of girls (which probably leads to the interventions being taken seriously and transforming attitudes). These mechanisms are more likely to be triggered when interventions involve single-gender sessions, provide opportunities for guided practice of skills and attitudes and focus on student relationships. We concluded that one reason why DRV perpetration effects tended to be greater among boys was that these interventions tended to do a good job of considering the gendered aspects of DRV, and acknowledged the disproportionate impacts of DRV on girls. This explanation also helped us to understand the ecological relationship between percentage of girls in the trial sample and reductions in DRV victimisation. Mechanisms are less likely to be triggered when interventions involve parent involvement or victim stories. The basic safety mechanism is more likely to generate reductions in DRV rather than GBV perpetration probably because of the more private nature of DRV, so that it is amenable to reduction via dating partners coming to view it as unacceptable. The more public nature of GBV probably means it is supported by peer social norms which are harder to modify.[227] Some interventions could prevent GBV but this is only likely to happen in high-income countries, where schools have more organisational capacity to implement actions which trigger the school transformation mechanism needed to reduce GBV.

Multi-component interventions aiming to trigger school transformation mechanism generally do not succeed in increasing student connections to school or changing social norms, and do not generate reductions in DRV/GBV. In some settings (schools with high capacity and resourcing in high-income countries), the school transformation mechanism (e.g. by interventions involving changes to school policies, student participation and/or school clubs) may be triggered and be sufficient to generate reductions in GBV. These CMOCs are summarised in Box 8.1.

These tested and refined CMOCs offer a number of insights about the potential for these school-based DRV/GBV interventions to be transferred to other populations and settings. For most schools in most settings, it may be less important to do something complex than to do something simple well, in order to prevent DRV. Under-resourced schools in areas of high deprivation may be best advised to focus on ensuring the basic safety of students by clamping down on abusive behaviours, postponing the encouragement of positive behaviours or the transformation of school social environments until they build the capacity to implement these well. School readiness, defined, for example, in terms of staff buy-in or strong school leadership, is likely to smooth the path to implementation. Engaging a critical mass of female students matters. In high-income countries and schools with high organisation capacity, it may be possible to reduce GBV using multi-component interventions to transform the school environment and student social norms.

Box 8.1 CMOCs for school-based prevention of DRV/GBV informed by synthesis of outcome evaluations

'Basic Safety' Mechanism of Benefit

Context: Particularly among boys and students with past involvement in DRV, and in schools with a critical mass of girls participating in intervention activities.

Mechanism: School staff deliver simple activities involving single-gender sessions, opportunities for guided practice of skills and attitudes and focusing on student relationships but not parent involvement or victim stories. These aim to prevent or stop DRV and GBV by encouraging students to develop knowledge and attitudes concerning the unacceptability of violence.

Outcome: Generating significant long-term reductions in DRV by promoting the motivations and capabilities needed to do this.

'Positive Development' Mechanism of Benefit

Context: Particularly in schools which lack the time, resources, leadership and commitment to deliver more difficult interventions.

Mechanism: School staff enact interventions involving single or multiple components aiming to develop students' positive development.

Outcome: Generating some long-term reductions in DRV via students developing capabilities and motivations going beyond merely the avoidance of violence to include, for example, conflict negotiation or maintaining healthy relationships.

'School Transformation' Mechanism of Benefit

Context: Only in schools in resource-rich settings which have the time, resources, leadership and commitment to deliver more difficult interventions.

Mechanism: Schools are transformed via changes to school policies, student participation and/or school clubs.

Outcome: Generating some long-term reductions in DRV and GBV.

8.4 Criticisms and Limitations of These Analytical Approaches

Reflecting on the methods we used in this review, our approach to using quantitative research to test our CMOCs might be open to criticism by some realist evaluators as taking a 'successionist' approach to causality.[61] But this would be a valid criticism only if we had examined associations between causes and effects without considering contextual contingencies. Instead, we believe we took a generative approach to understanding causality. We first developed a rich and contextual understanding of how mechanisms might generate different outcomes in different contexts, informed by engaging with intervention theories of change, broader theory and process evaluations as described in Chapter 7. We used this to develop CMOCs. We then tested whether these CMOCs aligned not just with narratives of results presented in studies but with contingent patterns of association in the empirical data that these studies reported.

We believe that this approach is no more successionist than the approaches used in more conventional realist reviews. This is because these realist reviews still rely on evidence from statistical analyses. It is just that these results are presented as narratives of causality (which rarely engage with contextual contingencies). Furthermore, the analyses we have described in this chapter draw not just on probabilistic statistical analyses of correlations but also on QCA, which allowed us to examine more complex combinations of conditions co-occurring with markers of outcomes.

Using these methods, it is possible for systematic reviews to develop more nuanced and useful conclusions than merely generating an estimate of the overall effect of an intervention on an outcome through pooling the effect estimates reported in included studies. The theories of change and process evaluations that we included in this and other reviews are often individually quite limited in scope and lacking in depth of analysis. However, our syntheses can bring together these studies in innovative ways to develop a far richer and more comprehensive analysis.

As we already mentioned in the section entitled 'Reviewing Mediation Analyses to Understand Mechanisms', compared to the quantitative analyses that we can do in our own trials, the analyses presented here are a lot more inductive than hypothetico-deductive in orientation. Some have more of a bearing on our CMOCs than others. This reflects not our changing our epistemological approach but rather that we have less control of what data we can collect in a systematic review because we are dependent on what analyses are reported in primary studies. Nonetheless, we hope we have demonstrated that it is still possible within a realist systematic review to conduct analyses drawing on included studies which can be used to reflect on and refine one's CMOCs. Our conclusions provide scientifically informative insights into the possible mechanisms by which school-based interventions can prevent DRV and GBV, and how these might be influenced by context. The broad searches, inclusion criteria and rigorous assessment of study quality ensured that we drew on evidence from a diversity of contexts but also that we were most informed by the strongest evidence. The question of which study designs to include in this type of review will depend on the intervention and population in question.

So far in this book, we have considered how evaluations and then systematic reviews can produce more scientifically rigorous and more useful evidence. In the remaining two chapters, we will explore how such evidence can be used by policymakers and practitioners (Chapter 9) and scientists (Chapter 10).

Chapter

9

Using Evidence to Inform Intervention Scale-Up and Transfer

The preceding chapters have explained how the use of realist approaches within evaluations and systematic reviews has the potential to offer much more nuanced information on how interventions work, and where and for whom they are likely to work best. This should help those policymakers or practitioners deciding whether to scale-up the interventions or those making decisions in other contexts about policy or practice to address complex health problems. But these policymakers or practitioners will need to review this evidence and then assess whether the interventions in question are likely to be a good fit for their settings and populations. This has only recently been an issue considered in the literature on evaluation and evidence-based policy.[234] In this chapter, we set out an approach which local policymakers or practitioners might use, again informed by realist approaches to evaluation. We suggest what forms of evidence and what local information such decision-makers might use.

9.1 Deciding to Implement an Intervention in a New Setting or Population

When considering whether to implement an intervention for which there is evidence from elsewhere of its effectiveness, local policymakers or practitioners will need to decide whether: it is such a good fit as to move to full implementation immediately; it looks like a promising intervention but with a need first for some local piloting and evaluation; or the intervention looks a poor fit, which is not worth pursuing. These are difficult and important decisions. Deciding to locally pilot and evaluate an intervention or deciding not to deliver it at all when it is in fact already 'good to go' will waste time and money. Potential beneficiaries will miss out on an effective intervention. An example of this scenario could be deciding to pilot a parenting intervention for child behavioural problems locally before any scale-up. The evidence suggests that these interventions have important benefits for parents and children across settings, and so may not need to be piloted when transferred to new settings.[53]

Deciding to go for immediate implementation of an intervention which is not yet quite fit for local purpose would also waste money and time, and could cause harm either directly or by displacing other, more effective interventions.[235] An example of this scenario might be youth work activities to prevent teenage pregnancy, which we saw in Chapter 1 have been found to be effective, ineffective or harmful in different settings.[10 11 236]

The key concept is uncertainty about whether an intervention generates benefits (sometimes known as 'equipoise').[237] We can apply this concept to interventions that have been evaluated elsewhere as effective and which are being considered for implementation in a new context. In this scenario, there is at least some remaining equipoise about whether the intervention will be more effective than whatever interventions constitute current, usual treatment in this new setting. So, any decision about piloting or implementation needs to consider what is current provision. Consideration also needs to attend to whether the intervention can be delivered feasibly and acceptably, reach potential beneficiaries and generate the intended outcomes in this new setting. Local decision-makers may also want to know about the size of impacts and the costs of intervention in the new setting to assess whether it is worth investing in. Hence, assessment of equipoise is not simple or easy. It involves multiple factors and involves questions of probability not binary distinctions. Decisions will undoubtedly need to be informed both by local information and by the results of previous evaluations of the intervention.

9.2 Applying a Realist Lens to Decisions about Local Implementation

To consider how local policymakers or practitioners should decide whether to proceed to full implementation, first pilot or not bother at all with a previously evaluated intervention, we consider the hypothetical example of a proposal for the implementation of a school-based social and emotional learning curriculum in US elementary schools previously evaluated as effective in promoting mental health across various settings.[238] By taking a realist approach to considering this situation, we will, as in previous chapters, be attending to questions of not merely what works, but also what works for whom and under what conditions.[61 75] We also take forward the understanding described in previous chapters that interventions provide resources that providers and beneficiaries use which may then trigger various mechanisms which may or may not generate outcomes. How intervention resources are used, the mechanisms that might be triggered and whether these generate outcomes will all vary between contexts. In the case of the social and emotional skills curriculum, it might be more feasible to deliver this in some schools and for some students than others. The mechanisms triggered, which involve students better understanding and managing their emotions and relationships with others, might be enough to generate mental health benefits in some settings but not others. The social and emotional skills curriculum is more likely to improve mental health for students who have needs (vulnerabilities) regarding these skills. For such students, these skill needs will play an important part in the 'aetiological mechanisms', that is those generating poor health. But it might not be so effective in settings where broader social factors, such as high rates of violence, are more important in these aetiological mechanisms. In considering this hypothetical case study, we first consider if the intervention was evaluated in contexts similar to the locality now being considered for implementation. Then we consider if the current context has the key features likely to be required for the intervention to be effective there.

9.3 Scenarios Where Intervention Transfer is Likely to be Successful

Implementation is likely to be most feasible and acceptable, and reach potential beneficiaries, in a new setting when two conditions are met.[2] Firstly, there is evidence that the intervention was feasible, acceptable and accessible from one or more existing process evaluations conducted in settings and with populations broadly similar to those present in the new setting (in terms of factors likely to affect implementation). These process evaluations will also ideally report on what factors supported implementation. In the case of social and emotional learning, there is evidence from a broad range of contexts that implementation is feasible and acceptable, and achieves reach. And there is evidence that implementation is promoted by school leaders championing the intervention, provision of staff training and good buy-in to the intervention among staff.[239] [240]

The second condition is that implementation in the new setting will be more likely successful when local information suggests that key factors enabling implementation are in place.[241] As well as the factors identified in previous evaluations, enabling factors might be identified from more general theories of what factors or processes promote good implementation.[66] [103] For example, the general theory of implementation suggests that successful implementation will be promoted via the presence of 'potential' (providers having the desire and ability needed for delivery); 'capability' (the intervention being workable and possible to integrate into existing services); 'contribution' (providers being able to make sense of the intervention, commit to its delivery, collaborate to make it work and reflect on progress); and 'capacity' (local structures, norms, roles and resources supporting implementation). Information on whether such factors are present locally might come from surveys or consultations with local practitioners, policymakers or communities; local audits of knowledge, skills, equipment and other resources possessed by providers; existing guidelines for practice; and evaluations or observations of local practice.[242] Some of this information will already exist but some might need to be newly collected as part of the needs assessment for the new intervention.

If implementation is considered possible, whether this will translate into effectiveness depends on two further factors. Firstly, it is more likely when the previous evaluations which reported the intervention was effective were several in number and used rigorous methods. If they are realist in orientation, such evaluations might also suggest how and for whom the intervention works. Individual studies might address such questions by reporting on qualitative evidence, mediation analyses or subgroup or moderation analyses, as discussed in chapters 4–6.[165] [241] Systematic reviews might provide useful evidence from subgroup analyses, meta-regression, network meta-analysis or qualitative comparative analysis, as discussed in chapters 7 and 8.[232] Existing evidence will ideally also indicate the size of effects, cost-effectiveness and any potential harms.

In the case of social and emotional learning, multiple studies have indeed reported that these interventions promote mental health, and mediation analyses have suggested that this occurs via improvements in social and emotional skills.[243] [244] Meta-regressions in systematic reviews suggest that benefits are most likely to occur in the USA (possibly because these interventions are well aligned with US culture) and with older elementary school students.[245] [246] There is also evidence that such interventions are cost-effective,[247] and do not harm (and in fact benefit) academic attainment.[248]

Secondly, we will be more confident that an intervention will generate benefits in a new setting if local information suggests that it will trigger its mechanisms of impact and these will generate the intended outcomes. Several factors can be considered to assess this. It will be more likely when the current usual treatment in the new setting is similar to that received by the control group in previous evaluations. It is also more likely when similar 'aetiological mechanisms' thought to generate the 'vulnerability' to the problems being targeted are operating in the new setting as with the sites of previous evaluations. This would ideally be assessed by comparing each setting in terms of the risk factors for the outcomes of interest.[8] [249] [250] In the case of social and emotional learning, this would mean comparing the original and new setting in terms of their prevalence of children's needs for improved social and emotional skills, and whether there is evidence that these are local risk factors for poor mental health.[251]

However, such evidence may not be available. The presence of similar aetiological mechanisms across settings might then instead need to be inferred based on socio-demographic similarities between the populations living in these settings. But this is not a fool proof strategy, for example, due to background changes and transitions in populations that may not be captured by cross-sectional comparisons between trial contexts and the new contexts. So we suggest that, when there are concerns that aetiological mechanisms might differ, this should be examined using local needs assessments. These should start with rapid qualitative assessments and involve new epidemiological assessments of risk factors if there is a high level of uncertainty.[252]

The Need for New Evaluations?

If the procedures in Section 9.3 suggest relatively low uncertainty about whether an intervention evaluated elsewhere as effective is a good fit for a new setting, it may nonetheless be wise to still evaluate it. The new evaluation might only need to evaluate process rather than outcomes. Aarons et al. have argued for 'borrowing strength' from earlier outcome evaluations to allow for evaluation in a new setting to focus only on process.[253] An example of this is an evaluation some of us did of the scale-up of the Intervention with Microfinance for AIDS and Gender Equity (IMAGE). As we have described in earlier chapters, the IMAGE intervention targeted women in poverty in rural South Africa and provided them with loans to start up small businesses, as well as education on gender and HIV, and enablement of campaigning on locally important issues. Following a cluster RCT trial which suggested that IMAGE was effective in reducing rates of intimate partner violence as well as sexual risk behaviour among family members,[4] it was scaled up to other rural areas in one region of South Africa.

Our evaluation of this scale-up aimed not to examine effectiveness but instead built on the process evaluation embedded within the cluster RCT to examine longer term implementation processes and potential mechanisms.[254] This new study suggested that the intervention was largely feasible and likely therefore to replicate the original benefits but that the campaigning component was often not sustainable, particularly when the women's poverty and social marginalisation undermined their ability to mount campaigns. This might suggest that this intervention be dropped in order to streamline the intervention in the new settings.

9.4 Scenarios Where Intervention Transfer is More Uncertain

Now we will consider some scenarios where local implementation of a previously evaluated intervention is less likely to be feasible or generate similar outcomes. The first such scenario is where there is uncertainty about implementation. It might be that the previous evaluations were not done in settings that resembled the new setting. Or they might have been conducted but identified barriers to implementation that are likely to present themselves in the new setting. Or they identified facilitators that are unlikely to be present in the new setting. Information from local consultations, surveys, audits, guidelines or observations might confirm that such factors present important barriers to delivery locally.

Let's again take school-based social and emotional skills interventions as an example. Consultations with heads or classroom teachers might suggest variable commitment to delivering the intervention. Audits of teachers' skills might indicate gaps. Analyses of school capacity might suggest staff lack the time, autonomy, resources and/or senior support to deliver the intervention. Observations might suggest that classrooms are too disrupted by student misbehaviour for good implementation.[218] These might suggest that, at the very least, it would be important to pilot the feasibility of delivery before any full implementation of social and emotional skills curricula is indicated. This piloting might try to address the potential barriers to implementation that have been identified to ensure the intervention has the best chance of being delivered properly. The local piloting will need to evaluate whether this is the case, by monitoring fidelity and/or using qualitative research to explore what factors affect feasibility. Local adaptations might be required.[7] [255]

In some circumstances, there might be even more profound uncertainty about whether the intervention is likely to be effective in the new setting. Firstly, there might be concerns that the intervention will not trigger the intended mechanisms. While the previous evaluations reported the intervention was effective, they might have been from settings or populations differing from those found locally. Or local information might suggest that the intervention will not trigger the intended mechanisms. In the case of school-based social and emotional education, consultations with teachers might indicate that classroom-based interactions won't trigger development of students' social and emotional skills because of concerns about students' attendance or engagement. Consultation with parents or students might suggest that the social and emotional skills which the intervention promotes do not align with local social norms.

Secondly, there may be concern that, even if triggered, the intervention mechanisms will not generate the intended outcomes. This might be of concern if there is local evidence that different aetiological mechanisms lie behind the mental health problems that the intervention is aiming to address. For example, surveys or routine data might suggest that prevalence of mental health problems among students is already low, that need for improved social and emotional skills is not common or that this need is not associated with mental health problems. Needs assessments might also suggest that, even if students do develop social and emotional skills, other local aetiological mechanisms might 'swamp' the intervention mechanisms. This might occur, for example, if there are high rates of local violence or child neglect or abuse. In such cases, intervention mechanisms may not disrupt the aetiological mechanisms causing children to have poor mental health. Where there are concerns but a lack of relevant evidence, there will be a need for new research. This might start with local consultations and then progress to local epidemiological studies if important uncertainties remain, and time and resources allow.

Where the concern is that intervention activities may not trigger mechanisms, this would suggest a need for a new effectiveness trial of the intervention adapted for local context. Local policymakers or practitioners would need to lobby research funders that this was a priority and/or lobby researchers so that these gained the funding to conduct the new study. Where the concern is that the intervention mechanisms, even if triggered, will not disrupt the local aetiological mechanisms or will be swamped by other aetiological mechanisms, then local decision-makers might decide that the intervention is simply not a good candidate and seek a different way to address the problem at hand.

9.5 Reflections

Our aim in this chapter has been to provide guidance for local policymakers and practitioners so they can assess whether to implement interventions previously evaluated elsewhere as effective. We have stressed the importance of assessing these existing evaluations not merely in terms of what they say about what works overall. Assessments of existing process evaluations should also consider how feasible, acceptable and accessible the intervention was, and what factors promoted this. Assessment of evaluations also needs to consider evidence of what worked for whom and how, drawing on qualitative, mediation, moderation, moderated mediation and/or qualitative comparative analyses within primary studies or systematic reviews. But we have also stressed the importance of decisions being informed by local needs assessment. Informed by realist evaluation, we provide two key insights into what is required of local needs assessments. Firstly, these should examine the local factors relating to the local potential, capability, contribution and capacity for implementation of the intervention. Such evidence will often not already exist and so new assessments will be needed. These might involve local consultations, surveys and audits. Secondly, where possible, local needs assessment should consider whether similar or different 'aetiological mechanisms' cause adverse outcomes in the new setting compared with those settings in which previous evaluations were conducted. This can be challenging to assess, ideally being based on epidemiological studies assessing the prevalence of local risk factors and how strongly these are associated with the outcomes of interest in the new setting versus the settings of the previous evaluations. Where there is not the time or money to conduct such research, similarities or differences in aetiological mechanisms might be inferred from similarities or differences in the socio-demographic profile of each population.

Major uncertainty as to whether an intervention can be feasibly, acceptably and accessibly implemented in a new setting suggests the need for local piloting to assess this. Where it is uncertain whether implementation will trigger the intended mechanisms, this suggests the need for a new trial of effectiveness. Where there are major doubts about whether the intervention mechanism, even if triggered, will generate the intended outcomes, this might indicate the need for local policymakers to look for different interventions to address the problem at hand in their setting.

It might sometimes be necessary to move rapidly to implementing an intervention in a new setting without firm evidence that it is locally appropriate. This might be the case when responding to humanitarian crises, epidemics and other emergencies.[256] In such cases, it should still be possible for some local assessments to be conducted at the same time that preparations are being made for delivery. These assessments could then inform refinements to the intervention as well as decisions about the extent and focus of monitoring and evaluation of the intervention.[257]

As well as thinking about whether an intervention is likely to be effective in a new setting, local decision-makers should also think through its likely impacts on health inequalities. Policymakers should similarly evaluate the match between their local contexts and intervention mechanisms to ensure that interventions are unlikely to exacerbate health inequalities. In the same way that evaluations should use clear, parsimonious theories to guide evaluations, decision-makers can use theories of health equity such as the social determinants of health theory,[258] to understand how access and uptake to intervention resources can impact health inequities. Importantly, these theories can also suggest intervention modifications to reduce the risk of equity harms or even to increase the possibility of equity benefits.

Limitations

One limitation with the approach we have set out here is that it is only applicable to situations in which there are previous evaluations about the intervention in question. There will, of course, be scenarios where there is no or very limited existing evaluation for an intervention being considered for implementation in a setting. In this situation, there is of course a much stronger argument for the need for new trials of effectiveness before any full implementation. In addition, while we have recognised that local policymakers' reading of the existing evaluation evidence should consider the size of effects, cost-effectiveness and the balance between benefits and harms, we have simplified our consideration of the various scenarios so these focus on more binary questions of whether interventions are effective or not.

The scenarios we have considered have also not addressed the question of harms and other unintended outcomes. We would recommend that reviews of existing evidence and local consultations also need to consider these as possibilities. Where these suggest that harms are considered substantial, likely and unavoidable, this would suggest the need to drop the intervention. Where they suggest that harms are a possibility but are less substantial in severity, less likely to occur and/or more avoidable, this might suggest that the intervention could still be a candidate but only after significant adaptation and then evaluation of effectiveness.[259] While our focus has been on complex health interventions and social or psychological mechanisms, biological systems are also complex and can vary across settings and populations, so the framework we offer here might also apply to biomedical interventions, especially in an era of personalised medicine.[260]

9.6 Conclusion

This chapter has considered how evaluation evidence might be used by policymakers or practitioners when making decisions about what interventions to deliver in a local setting. The next chapter stays with the topic of how evaluation evidence might be used but considers how scientists might use evaluation evidence to refine their theories about the world.

10 Using Evidence to Refine Middle Range Theory

10.1 Limits to the Direct Use of Evaluation Evidence

Evaluation evidence is useful for informing decisions about implementing specific interventions in sites beyond those it is initially evaluated within, as discussed in the previous chapter. For example, a cluster trial of the 'ASSIST' peer-education intervention in schools to prevent smoking found that this was effective.[86] The trial was useful in providing evidence for public health and education policymakers as well as schools, indicating that ASSIST was a potentially effective means to prevent smoking.[261] However, over time, evaluation evidence becomes gradually less useful for directly informing decisions about which intervention to implement. This is because things inevitably change so that the context within which the intervention was implemented and evaluated no longer resembles contexts where policymakers and practitioners are making decisions about what interventions to deliver. For example, in the case of the ASSIST intervention, over time schools and the education system within which they operate will evolve, as will youth culture and the aetiological mechanisms generating smoking among adolescents. Peer norms might become less important influences on smoking compared to other determinants. This means that we can be less and less confident that any new implementation of the ASSIST intervention will involve similar processes of delivery or receipt, or similar mechanisms of impact. The specific intervention, in this case ASSIST, might wane in its feasibility and acceptability and become less effective. The specific form of the various components may need to be updated to trigger the intended mechanisms. Or the entire intervention might need to be more drastically modified to trigger different mechanisms. New evaluations will be needed to evaluate these processes and mechanisms.

Evaluation evidence is also less useful for directly informing decisions about which intervention to implement if we are considering a very different geographical setting. This is also true when the decision about what intervention to implement concerns a slightly different sort of intervention or outcome. Evidence from the ASSIST intervention study would, for example, not be able to directly inform decisions about smoking prevention in schools in a low-income country. It would be of even less direct use when informing decisions about physician-led smoking prevention interventions or interventions aiming to reduce use of other substances, regardless of when or where these were to be delivered.

10.2 Broader Uses of Evidence

But this does not mean that evaluations cannot have a broader and enduring value beyond informing immediate decisions about implementing similar interventions for similar outcomes in similar settings.[262] In this chapter, we argue that a critically important but highly

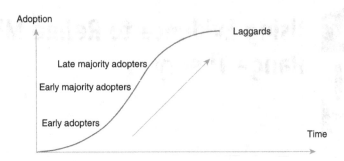

Figure 10.1 Diffusion of innovations theory

underappreciated use of evaluation evidence is in contributing to the testing and refinement of scientific theory. A broader and more enduring value of the ASSIST trial[263] might be in its contribution to theory.

For example, the ASSIST trial findings provide support for Everett Rogers' theory of the 'diffusion of innovations' and provide useful refinements to how this theory might be applied to diffusing health messages through adolescent social networks.[264] This theory proposes that 'innovations' (new products, behaviours or ideas) diffuse through a social network of people via an S-shaped curve (Figure 10.1). Early adoption rates are slow because 'early adopters', who are especially drawn to the innovation, are unlikely to be typical or well-connected members of the network. But it speeds up as adoption eventually reaches the 'early majority', who are somewhat less immediately drawn to the innovation but then transmit it more rapidly because they are more influential and better connected. It gets even faster as adoption spreads to 'late majority' adopters, who are even less immediately drawn to the innovation but transmit it rapidly once adopted because of their strong influence and connections. Adoption rates then slow again as the only people left are 'laggards', who are the least well-disposed towards the innovation and also not very influential or well-connected within the network.

What the ASSIST study told us was, first, that the diffusion of innovations could be used to inform a peer-education intervention that treated an anti-smoking message as the innovation and, second, that adoption rates could be accelerated by ensuring that influential and well-connected young people were targeted to be the early adopters and transmitters of this innovation. This insight might help inform decisions about the implementation of various social interventions over greater stretches of time, geography, intervention types or outcomes than merely school-based prevention of smoking in high-income countries around the turn of the twenty-first century.

The contribution of evaluations to advancing broader scientific theory is more than of academic interest because it is such theory which then informs the next generation of interventions. A clear example of using scientific theory to inform interventions is provided by Covid communications. In the early days of the Covid-19 pandemic in 2020, some of us were involved in advising the UK government on how to encourage the population to adhere to restrictions aiming to prevent transmission. Communications interventions had to be developed rapidly and could not be informed directly by empirical evidence from intervention studies given the novelty of the virus and the need for unprecedented and rapid behaviour change to reduce the spread of the infection.[265] However, despite this lack of direct empirical evidence, a body of behavioural science did exist which we used to advise on the development of communication interventions. This body of scientific theory had been developed through the study of other infections (including other coronaviruses such as 'MERS' and 'SARS') as well as other areas of health and even other areas of social behaviour (such as the study of crowd behaviour).

This scientific theory suggested a number of principles which were used to help ensure that the communications interventions deployed were more likely to achieve their intended outcomes and less likely to generate harmful unintended consequences.[266] For example, we drew on social identity theory to recommend that 'protect each other' messages were more likely to encourage people to adhere to the restrictions than 'protect yourself' messages.[267] Similarly, we drew on social influence theory[268] and moral foundations of behaviour theory,[269] for which there was some evidence of informing effective interventions in other areas of health.[270 271]

Using scientific theory to inform interventions and using evaluations to inform scientific theory aligns with realist principles. Realists view the results of empirical research being transferable not in terms of statistical generalisability but rather in terms of analytic generalisability. Whereas the former asks, 'can we expect the same size effect as we saw before in a new but similar sample?', the latter asks, 'does our understanding of the mechanisms by which an intervention generates outcomes help us in a new context?'

What, then, is scientific theory? When thinking about complex health interventions and the sorts of problems they address, we are interested in theory about social mechanisms. As we saw in Chapter 4, the theory concerned with how such mechanisms operate is sometimes referred to within social science as 'middle range theory'.[26] This theory is about the general mechanisms, not necessarily triggered by a particular intervention, which generate outcomes. It is analytically generalisable enough to apply to a range of contexts or outcomes, but specific enough to still be useful when applied to a specific empirical case. So it is different to theory of change, which concerns the mechanisms triggered by a specific intervention. In Chapter 4, we described how theories of change were first popularised by Carol Weiss and others[2 106] and how realist evaluators and others have improved how we think about theory of change by proposing that these need to engage with how mechanisms interact with context to generate outcomes.[61 111]

10.3 How Evaluations Can Inform Theories

So how might evaluations of complex health interventions contribute towards the testing and refinement of middle range theory? Let's first of all think about the more general question of how empirical research can contribute to testing and refining theory. In proposing his 'hypothetico-deductive' approach to science, Karl Popper argued that experiments should aim to falsify hypotheses, which are derived from theory.[272] Hypotheses are empirically testable predictions about specific mechanisms in specific circumstances. In this approach, scientific knowledge consists of those theories that are in principle falsifiable, have been subject to experimental tests and have not yet been falsified. Where hypotheses are falsified, the theories from which they were derived need to be abandoned or refined so they can be further tested.

Popper presented the hypothetico-deductive approach as an alternative to the empiricist view, which we discussed in Chapter 3. This presents scientific knowledge as being built up, bottom-up from scientific observation. Popper, among others, judged that such an 'inductive' approach to science is unsound because no number of empirical observations (e.g. that all the swans that we have observed are white) will allow the construction of a general theory (e.g. that all swans are white). This is because there remains the possibility of disconfirming evidence (e.g. an observed black swan).[272] Popper also thought induction was inadequate as a basis for building scientific theory because if they did not have some starting theory, scientists would not know what to observe. And Popper also argued that scientific theories need to specify the contingencies that underpin theorised mechanisms, with no mechanisms generating the same effects in all contexts.[25]

Critical realists, such as Roy Bhaskar, and realist evaluators, such as Ray Pawson and Nick Tilley, accept the basic argument that science should be oriented towards testing hypotheses derived from theory. However, they contend that empirical tests rarely provide a basis for the falsification of theory.[61][74] As we saw in Chapter 3, realists argue that causal mechanisms in the realm of the real generate observable events in the realm of the actual which may be observed in the realm of the empirical. But they will do so differently in different contexts because of variation in what other mechanisms operate in these contexts. Therefore, if a mechanism does not generate observed events as hypothesised, this may be because it lacked the contexts with which it needed to interact to generate outcomes or it was swamped by other mechanisms operating in that context. So a failure of observed events to live up to what a hypothesis promised does not mean that the theory has to be abandoned. Instead, it may mean that the theory needs to be refined so that it can better specify the contexts in which the mechanism will generate the expected outcome.[61] This position is actually not very different to Popper's idea that scientific theories need to specify the contingencies that underpin mechanisms.[25]

Let's now consider the specific case of trials and middle range theory. Trials are oriented towards testing the theory of change for that intervention.[39] Where the theory of change is informed by a middle range theory, perhaps the evaluation could also be useful for testing the middle range theory. Pawson and Tilley have recommended using middle range theories to inform CMOCs.[61] But neither they nor those advocating theory-based evaluation have argued for evaluation to be used to test and refine middle range theory.[273] We think this is a missed opportunity.

Consider the hypothetical example of an intervention being subject to evaluation which uses an appropriate design and methods to minimise bias and confounding, and optimises statistical power. The intervention is delivered as planned and reaches the intended potential beneficiaries who find it acceptable. The evaluation finds, however, that the intervention does not generate the intended outcomes as described by its theory of change. It might be that the overall result is null or that the outcomes expected for a particular subgroup do not manifest. Such results would suggest that the theory of change for the intervention might be incorrect, particularly if other studies tell a similar story. This might lead the evaluators to believe that the choice of the middle range theory to inform the intervention theory of change in the first place was not great. Maybe another middle range theory could have suggested a different intervention theory of change, which had the potential to generate the outcomes in question in that particular context.

But we think this evaluation might offer some additional insights. It might imply that the hypothesised mechanism does not generate the expected outcomes in the context in which the evaluation occurred. This might inform refinement of the middle range theory so that it includes the contextual contingencies under which the theorised mechanism does and does not generate outcomes. If we have several different studies done in different contexts, these might help refine the middle range theory. Multiple such studies, some with null results and some with more positive results, could contribute to the gradual refinement of this middle range theory so that it comes to comprehensively include contextual contingencies. This is potentially of great value in making sure that middle range theories are more attentive to the contextual contingencies which realists and Popperians both recognise as important.[25 74]

We have argued in this book that the best way for evaluations to provide information about the likely transferability of a particular intervention is for evaluations to test and refine an intervention's theory of change and CMOC.[55 238] But this only enables one to understand the likely transferability of that particular intervention. Another, complementary, approach would be for evaluations to also inform refinement of middle range theory. The refined middle range theory could then be used to make predictions about the likely transferability not just of a particular intervention but also of a broader category of intervention, aiming to trigger broadly similar mechanisms but using different intervention methods to do so.[274] This would be particularly powerful when there are multiple studies from different contexts to inform refinements to middle range theory.

We can illustrate this through some of our own works. As discussed in previous chapters, we are interested in using the theory of human functioning and school organisation to inform health interventions in schools. To recap, this theory proposes that we can reduce student involvement in health-related risk behaviours by promoting their commitment to school: to the school's 'instructional' (i.e. teaching and learning) and 'regulatory' (i.e. discipline and community) orders. This first requires that schools 'reframe' provision so that this aligns with students' needs and 're-classify' school processes so that they erode various 'boundaries' between staff and students, students' academic and broader personal development and the culture of the school and its local community. The theory suggests that these mechanisms will be particularly beneficial for more disadvantaged students, for whom commitment to school is often not the default.

Our trial of Learning Together and our systematic review of school-based interventions to prevent DRV and GBV suggested various ways in which this middle range theory might be refined. For example, the Learning Together trial suggested that the theorised mechanisms might not particularly benefit disadvantaged students and that it might only be possible to bring about reframing and reclassification in schools possessing the sort of culture that would encourage staff to want to achieve such changes, and the organisational capacity to do so. And our systematic review of DRV/GBV prevention in schools suggested that some boundaries might actually be health promoting so that the theory needed to be clearer as to which boundaries should be eroded and why. Some of us have also previously conducted a systematic review of interventions which aimed to deliver health education integrated with academic education to prevent violence and substance use. This reported that such interventions are effective in preventing adolescent substance use but not violence.[222] This might suggest that the theory of human functioning and school organisation might need to specify which aspects of boundary erosion are most important for generating which health outcomes.

10.4 Barriers to Using Evaluation to Inform Refinement of Theory

However, this use of evaluation studies to reflect on and refine middle range theory is currently not happening much. The way that trials and other evaluations of complex health interventions are currently designed means that these cannot always easily be used to test and refine middle range theory. There are several challenges.

Multiple Theories

The first is that not many evaluations focus on an intervention informed by a single middle range theory. Many interventions have multiple components and aim to trigger multiple mechanisms. They have a theory of change informed by multiple middle range theories. In terms of potential impact this is, of course, likely to be generally positive. Such interventions will generally be more effective and more likely to transfer successfully across contexts. Their multiple mechanisms are more likely to address diverse population needs within and across contexts.[127] The evaluations of such interventions might be useful in understanding how these different intervention components and mechanisms interact with each other.[259] However, evaluations of such interventions don't provide a very neat way of testing any one middle range theory. If the evaluation reports that the intervention is ineffective, it is not clear what this tells us about the various different middle range theories informing the intervention.

For example, some of us conducted a systematic review of e-health interventions for men who have sex with men to prevent sexual risk and substance use and promote mental health.[224] E-health interventions refer to those delivered via apps or other software on smart phones or other electronic equipment. They offer an interactional means by which people can learn about a health topic and apply this to their everyday lives, often involving a way for people to monitor their behaviour and assess whether this aligns with their goals.

Several interventions in our review had theories of change drawing on more than one middle range theory.[224] For example, the 'Hot and Safe M4M' intervention drew on the information motivation behaviour (IMB) model and on motivational interviewing theory.[275] The IMB model proposes that behaviour change can be generated by providing information, developing skills and modifying motivation related to the behaviour in question.[276] Motivational interviewing theory proposes that individuals contemplating behaviour change will be at different stages in terms of motivation and that interventions need to help individuals at each stage resolve their uncertainties and build motivation.[277]

Another intervention included in our review was the 'TXT-Auto' intervention. This was informed by social cognitive theory and the health belief model.[278] Social cognitive theory proposes that individuals can acquire knowledge or skills by observing others during social interactions.[279] The health belief model postulates that behaviour change comes about via people changing their beliefs about a health problem, their perceptions of the benefits of action, their perceptions of barriers to action and their self-efficacy to initiate change.[280]

Both Hot and Safe M4M and TXT-Auto were found ineffective in reducing sexual risk behaviours.[281] This suggests that the intervention theories of change were not supported (at least in these evaluation contexts) but it is not clear what the trials tell us about the validity of the various middle range theories informing the interventions' theories of change. Perhaps the 'Hot and Safe M4M' intervention was ineffective because, for the population and outcome in the trial, information, motivation and/or behavioural skills were not key influences on behaviour. Or perhaps for the population and outcome in question, behaviour change was hindered by trying to focus the intervention on participants' varying levels of motivation. It is difficult to say because the intervention theories of change were informed by more than one middle range theory with no explanation of how these theories were integrated to inform a single intervention.

Unclear Theoretical Constructs

The second problem with using trials of complex health interventions to shed light on middle range theory is that some middle range theories do not describe their constructs with enough clarity that they can be empirically tested. One example is the lack of clarity within the theory of human functioning and school organisation about which boundaries in schools are healthy and which are unhealthy, which we highlighted in our systematic review of school-based interventions to prevent DRV and GBV.[282] This theory proposes that schools can promote health by increasing students' commitment to school. One way that it theorises how schools can achieve this is by eroding 'boundaries', including those between staff and students, and between the school and its community. However, in the course of the synthesis, we realised that this consideration of boundaries was not clear enough. There was a suggestion in some of the theories of change in studies we included in the review that some boundaries actually contributed to students' well-being. For example, some student–teacher boundaries were theorised as being useful in maintaining staff authority to challenge student violence. Some boundaries between schools and communities were theorised as helping prevent violence at school when the schools were in tough neighbourhoods with social norms supportive of gender-based violence. We came to see that the theory of human functioning and school organisation wasn't clear enough in how it defined an 'unhealthy' versus a 'healthy' boundary.

Unclear Inter-relationships between Constructs

A third problem is that many middle range theories are difficult to test because it is not clear exactly what the relationships between the constructs in the theory are. For example, it is not clear whether the IMB model is proposing that for an *individual* to change their behaviour, they must increase their level of information, skills *and* motivation, or instead they just need to increase *any one* of these. Or perhaps the IMB model is proposing that increasing any one of these three constructs will change behaviour contingent on the other two having already reached a certain threshold. The theory might be suggesting that, to achieve population-level behaviour change, an intervention must increase *every person's* information, skills *and* motivation. Or it might be suggesting that population change can be achieved by increasing some people's information, some people's skills and some people's motivation. This might seem like typical academic pedantry but we think these questions are important to clarify if we are going to be able to design evaluations to test middle range theory and then interpret their results.

Too Many Constructs

A final problem is that some middle range theories include so many constructs that are theorised to influence an outcome that it makes them difficult to test. For example, we did a systematic review of evaluations of interventions aiming to modify school environments to reduce substance use and violence. The theories of change for some interventions were informed by middle range theories proposing that a young person's health or development is influenced by multiple factors at different social levels.[283] For example, the 'Cyber Friendly Schools' intervention was informed by ecological systems theory.[284] This theory proposes that child development is influenced by mechanisms operating at the level of the microsystem (the institutions and groups with which the child interacts); mesosystems (the interconnections between these microsystems); the exosystem (the links between social settings directly involving the child and those that don't); the macrosystem (the overarching culture); and the chronosystem (broader environmental events and transitions, and changing socio-historical circumstances).[285]

It is clear that, as well as some of these constructs being vague, there were simply a lot of them. The 'Cyber Friendly Schools' intervention aimed to increase family awareness of cyberbullying and modify school organisational structures to reduce cyberbullying, with families and schools being theorised as miscrosystems. A trial of the intervention reported no effects on violence.[284] This evidence can tell us nothing about the validity of ecological systems theory because it only engaged with one of the theory's many levels.

The more explanatory constructs a theory includes, the more difficult it will be for any empirical study to test the theory's validity in predicting an outcome. Putting aside our reflection on the vagueness of how the relationships between constructs are described in the IMB model, it is possible to imagine an empirical study examining whether increasing people's level of information, skills and motivation are associated with changes in behaviour. This could be done with a trial comparing an intervention with a control condition where the intervention aimed to increase information, skills and motivation, and the evaluation assessed changes in measures of these constructs as well as changes in the behaviour in question. In theory, the strongest design would be a study with multiple intervention arms aiming to increase various combinations of information, skills and motivation. In practice, such a study would be unwieldy, but such a study would be even more challenging if applied to testing theories with more explanatory constructs, such as ecological systems theory. Theories such as ecologic systems theory, which include many explanatory factors, may be useful as 'omnibus theories', summarising our ideas or knowledge about the overall range of factors affecting health or human development. But they are not useful as 'working theories', which suggests hypotheses open to empirical testing.

10.5 How to Make Evaluations More Useful for Refining Theory

We have several suggestions to make trials of complex health interventions better able to contribute towards testing and refinement of middle range theory.

Proof of Principle Studies

Our first suggestion is that there could be some investment in 'proof of principle' studies. These would focus on interventions with a single mechanism informed by a single middle range theory. For example, one might construct a proof of principle study to test whether men who have sex with men who engage with an online intervention to promote motivation to reduce substance use actually do report increases in motivation and reductions in substance use. The intervention would focus on a single mechanism but it could still involve multiple intervention activities if these all aimed to promote motivation. The intervention could, for example, aim to build motivation via sharing testimonies from other men who have changed their behaviour, or by asking the men to complete self-assessments of how much they use substances, and how this sits with their broader life goals.

Such proof of principle studies would sometimes be done in preparation for pragmatic evaluations of scalable interventions. They would help us understand how specific intervention mechanisms generate certain outcomes before putting together a pragmatic intervention aiming to trigger several such mechanisms to achieve a significant health impact. Such studies would be an occasional complement to pragmatic evaluations of multi-mechanism, multi-component interventions, rather than a complete alternative. A complementary programme of proof of principle and pragmatic evaluations would help us determine whether impacts can be achieved by parsimonious, single-theory interventions and which arise only through the action of multiple mechanisms triggered by complex, multi-theory interventions. Even where such proof of principle studies are not run, it might still be possible for some pragmatic evaluations to provide some insights in the validity of middle range theory. We hope our various studies which examine the theory of human functioning and school organisation are an example of this.

Focus on Theories with Clear Constructs

Our second suggestion is that those using middle range theory to develop intervention theories of change should concentrate on those middle range theories which have clearly defined constructs. This should help ensure that, when evaluations come to assess these theories of change, it will be possible to determine if the theorised mechanisms have been triggered. Some middle range theories, such as the IMB model and social cognitive theory, do clearly define their constructs.

This seems to be more common in psychology and economics than in sociology or anthropology. One factor might be that many sociological and anthropological theories are not really middle range theories at all. They don't aim to predict causal relationships between phenomena but instead aim to explore the informal rules of social institutions, describe social phenomena or provide an interpretive lens.[286][287] But there also seems to be a tendency in sociology and anthropology for theories to consider causal relationships but to do so without using clear or consistent terminology to define their terms. It has been suggested that this results in some ostensibly divergent sociological theories actually having significant but undeclared overlaps.[288] There have been attempts to systematise sociological theories so that they are better suited to being tested and refined through empirical research.[288] Such efforts might usefully be applied to complex health intervention research because sociological and anthropological theory should have a key role in informing complex health interventions involving social mechanisms not reducible to psychology or economics.[13] Where middle range theories include vague constructs (or where it is not clear how constructs are causally related to one another), they should be refined to make them clearer prior to empirical testing.

Focus on Parsimonious Theories

Our final suggestion is that theories of change should be informed by middle range theories that are parsimonious: limited in how many causal factors they include. This could advance scientific understanding by ensuring that evaluations might help test and refine middle range theory. In turn, this should improve the validity of our stock of middle range theories. This should then be useful in providing broader understanding of what mechanisms can generate what outcomes in what contexts. Such understanding should then inform the theories of change for future interventions.

Where Necessary, Use Retroduction

In some cases, there may not be an obvious choice of theory, even in the light of accumulated evidence about intervention effectiveness and functioning. In this case, retroduction can be a useful tool. Retroduction is working backwards from a pattern of results to theorise, based on all the evidence at our disposal, why some interventions may have been more effective than others. The credibility of retroduction relies on researchers' ability to demonstrate the trustworthiness of their analysis. For example, was there cherry-picking? Or did researchers discount negative results without good reason? In our experience, retroduction is most useful in systematic reviews that precede trials. It may also be the case that there is an 'emergent fit' between explanations generated by retroduction and a clear, parsimonious theory.

Conclusion

This book has argued that evaluation is important to ensure that complex health interventions (i.e. those with multiple components interacting with each other and with the context of delivery) are effective in achieving their intended outcomes, represent good value for money and cause minimal harm. It makes the case that randomised controlled trials represent the most scientifically rigorous means of assessing the outcomes of interventions. By having a control group, they enable the 'signal' of intervention effects to be distinguished analytically from the 'noise' of other trends and influences. By having randomised allocation to intervention and control groups, they allow as fair a comparison as possible. We argued that, in doing so, trials do not attempt to ignore context but rather they take proper account of it. Effect estimates represent not the isolated impact of an intervention but rather the value-added provided, in interaction with all the other influences on an outcome present within a context.

However, we went on to argue that, currently, most trials and systematic reviews are not as scientific or useful as they could be. Trials generally focus on carefully estimating quantitative effect estimates, often failing to adequately explore the mechanisms through which interventions actually work or how these interact with context to generate different outcomes in different settings or with different populations. Many trials also fail to contribute to the development, testing and refinement of scientific theory about these mechanisms. Systematic reviews concentrate on pooling effect estimates from multiple trials from different contexts as though there was one underlying effect, or distribution of effect, across contexts that can be uncovered by meta-analysis. They often, like most trials, fail to examine mechanisms and how these might interact with context to generate different outcomes in different settings and populations. We argued that these omissions are not merely of scientific concern. They hinder trials and systematic reviews in their role of providing useful evidence for understanding which interventions are likely to be the most promising candidates for transfer to other settings and with other populations.

We examined the realist critique of, and proposed alternative to, trials and systematic reviews. We accepted realist arguments that interventions need to be evaluated in terms of the mechanisms they trigger and how these interact with context to generate different outcomes in different settings and with different populations. We welcomed the realist approach to constructing hypotheses to be tested in evaluations in terms of CMOCs. But we were not persuaded by realist arguments that randomised trials are not a proper scientific design or that it is better to test these CMOCs using observational designs which do not use randomisation.

We disagreed with some realist evaluators' view that trials cannot be used within realist evaluation because they cannot encompass the diversity of contexts needed to test CMOCs and because they are irretrievably positivist and so inimical to realist enquiry. We argued that trials do not of necessity embody a positivist approach to the science of complex health interventions. They take a hypothetico-deductive, not an inductive, empiricist approach to scientific knowledge. They can examine hypotheses derived from scientific theories which attend to the deep mechanisms through which outcomes are generated. And when applied to understanding social mechanisms, they use very different methods to trials used in the natural sciences, such as agriculture and pharmacology. We also argued that systematic reviews provide the least biased means of assessing the evidence base in order to draw general conclusions about intervention impacts.

We went on to demonstrate how our own trial of the Learning Together whole-school intervention to prevent bullying set out to define, refine and test CMOCs. We showed in detail how middle range theory, previous research and public consultation were used to define CMOCs. We then showed how qualitative research conducted as part of process evaluation was used to refine these CMOCs. Then we demonstrated how a range of different quantitative methods done as part of the trial were used to test and so further refine the CMOCs.

We also disagreed with realist evaluators that to examine CMOCs, reviews of evidence need to abandon systematic methods. We identified the limitations of realist reviews in terms of their non-comprehensive searches, lack of attention to study quality and synthesis of outcome findings in terms of narratives rather than quantitative regularities. We presented our own systematic review of school-based prevention of dating and relationship violence and gender-based violence as an example of another way to examine realist questions while still using systematic methods of searching, quality appraisal and synthesis. We demonstrated how CMOCs could be defined ('tracked') through synthesis of intervention descriptions and theories of change; how these CMOCs could be refined through synthesis of process evaluations; and then tested through various quantitative outcome syntheses. We demonstrated how our findings from both this trial and this systematic review offered more scientifically interesting and more useful findings.

We then went on to show how policymakers and practitioners in settings beyond the sites of evaluation might make use of evidence from realist trials and systematic reviews as well as local needs assessment to identify the best candidate interventions for their local contexts and decide whether such interventions could be delivered immediately at scale or instead first required local evaluation of processes or even of outcomes. Finally, we reflected on how evidence from realist trials and systematic reviews might be of value not only in drawing conclusions about specific interventions and their theories of change but also in testing and refining the middle range theories which inform these interventions. We argued that, while evaluation evidence would be of most immediate use in informing decisions about the implementation of the specific interventions being evaluated, a broader and more enduring use for evaluation could be in suggesting refinements to middle range theory. Such refinements might then be used to inform and influence the next generation of complex health interventions.

Thus, we have set out a method by which evaluation can become more useful by becoming more scientific and moving beyond being a form of sophisticated descriptive monitoring of 'what works'. Evaluation can become more scientific both by continuing to use the most scientifically rigorous methods, and by being focused on the testing and refining of scientific theory. Critical realism and realist evaluation approaches offer a useful framework for constructing such theory because they offer the most plausible account of how causality operates in the complex social world. We hope that, by making these arguments, we have persuaded readers that trials and systematic reviews need to be reoriented and reformed rather than thrown away altogether. The incorporation of realist enquiry methods into randomised trials and systematic reviews offers us the best hope of evaluation and evidence synthesis that generate evidence which is both more scientific and more useful.

References

1. Skivington K, Matthews L, Simpson SA, et al. A new framework for developing and evaluating complex interventions: Update of Medical Research Council guidance. *British Medical Journal* 2021;30(374):n2061.

2. Moore G, Audrey S, Barker M, et al. *Process Evaluation of Complex Interventions: UK Medical Research Council (MRC) Guidance.* London: MRC Population Health Science Research Network 2014.

3. Medical Research Council. *A Framework for the Development and Evaluation of Randomised Controlled Trials for Complex Interventions to Improve Health.* London: MRC 2000.

4. Pronyk PM, Hargreaves JR, Kim JC, et al. Effect of a structural intervention for the prevention of intimate-partner violence and HIV in rural South Africa: A cluster randomised trial. *Lancet* 2006;368(9551):1973–83.

5. Hargreaves J, Hatcher A, Strange V, et al. Process evaluation of the Intervention with Microfinance for AIDS and Gender Equity (IMAGE) in rural South Africa. *Health Education Research* 2010;25(1):27–40. https://doi.org/10.1093/her/cyp054.

6. Nielsen JH, Melendez-Torres GJ, Rotevatn TA, et al. How do reminder systems in follow-up screening for women with previous gestational diabetes work?: A realist review. *BMC Health Services Research* 2021;21(1):535. https://doi.org/10.1186/s12913-021-06569-z.

7. Hawe P, Shiell A, Riley T. Complex interventions: How 'out of control' can a randomised controlled trial be? *British Medical Journal* 2004;328:1561–63.

8. Bonell C, Oakley A, Hargreaves J, et al. Trials of health interventions and empirical assessment of generalizability: Suggested framework and systematic review. *British Medical Journal* 2006;333:346–49.

9. Kirby DB, Rhodes T, Campe S. *Implementation of Multi-component Youth Programs to Prevent Teen Pregnancy Modelled after the Children's AID Society: Carrera Program.* Scotts Valley CA: ETR Associates 2005.

10. Philiber S, Kaye JW, Herrling S. *The National Evaluation of the Children's Aid Society Carrera Model Program to Prevent Teen Pregnancy.* New York: Philiber Research Associations 2001.

11. Wiggins M, Bonell C, Sawtell M, et al. Health outcomes of youth development programme in England: Prospective matched comparison study. *British Medical Journal* 2009;339:b2534.

12. Dishion TJ, McCord J, Poulin F. When interventions harm. *American Psychologist* 1999;54(9):755–64.

13. Hawe P, Shiell A, Riley T. Theorising interventions as events in systems. *American Journal of Community Psychology* 2009;43(3–4):267–76.

14. Sacks H, Chalmers TC, Smith HJ. Randomized versus historical controls for clinical trials. *American Journal of Medicine* 1982;72:233–40.

15. Hooker W. *Physician and Patient.* New York: Baker and Scribner 1847.

16. Hawe P, Shiell A, Riley T. Theorising interventions as events in systems. *American Journal of Community Psychology* 2009;43(3–4):267–76.

17. Lorenc T, Oliver K. Adverse effects of public health interventions: A conceptual framework. *Journal of Epidemiology Community Health* 2014;68(3):288–90.

18. Killeen T, Hien D, Campbell A, et al. Adverse events in an integrated trauma-focused intervention for women in community substance abuse treatment. *Journal of Substance Abuse Treatment* 2008;35:304–11.

19. Gould MS, Marrocco FA, Kleinman M, et al. Evaluating iatrogenic risk of youth suicide screening programs: A randomized controlled trial. *Journal of American Medical Association* 2005;**293**:1635–43.

20. Smith SW, Hauben M, Aronson JK. Paradoxical and bidirectional drug effects. *Drug Safety* 2012;**35**(3):173–89.

21. Lorenc T, Petticrew M, Welch V, et al. What types of interventions generate inequalities? Evidence from systematic reviews. *Journal of Epidemiology and Community Health* 2013;**67**(2):190–93. https://doi.org/10.1136/jech-2012-201257.

22. Thomson H, Hoskins R, Petticrew M, et al. Evaluating the health effects of social interventions. *British Medical Journal* 2004;**328**:282–85.

23. Ross D, Wight D. The role of randomized controlled trials in assessing sexual health interventions. In: Stephenson J, Imrie J, Bonell C, eds. *Effective Sexual Health Interventions: Issues in Experimental Evaluation.* Oxford: Oxford University Press 2003:35–48.

24. Campbell DT. Methods for the experimenting society. *American Journal of Evaluation* 1991;**12**(3):223–60.

25. Popper K. *The Poverty of Historicism.* London: Routledge & Kegan Paul 1957.

26. Merton RK. *Social Theory and Social Structure.* New York: Free Press 1968.

27. Jay D. *The Socialist Case.* London: Faber & Faber 1938.

28. Campbell DT, Russo JJ. *Social Experimentation.* Thousand Oaks, CA: SAGE 1999.

29. Lister R. New labour: A study in ambiguity from a position of ambivalence. *Critical Social Policy* 2001;**21**(4):425–47.

30. Mykhalovskiy E, Weir L. The problem of evidence-based medicine: Directions for social science. *Social Science & Medicine* 2004;**59**:1059–69.

31. Robertson A. Shifting discourses on health in Canada: From health promotion to population health. *Health Promotion International* 1998;**13**(2):155–66.

32. Wildgen A, Denny K. Health equity's missing substance: (Re)Engaging the normative in public health discourse and knowledge making. *Public Health Ethics* 2020;**13**(3):247–58.

33. Schrecker T. Can health equity survive epidemiology? Standards of proof and social determinants of health. *Preventive Medicine* 2013;**57**(6):741–44.

34. Parker RG, Easton D, Klein CH. Structural barriers and facilitators in HIV prevention: A review of international research. *AIDS* 2000;**14**(Suppl 1):S22–32.

35. Blankenship KM, Reinhard E, Sherman SG, et al. Structural interventions for HIV prevention among women who use drugs: A global perspective. *Journal of Acquired Immune Deficiency Syndrome* 2015;**69**(Suppl 2):S140–45. https://doi.org/10.1097/qai.0000000000000638.

36. Cohn S, Clinch M, Bunn C, et al. Entangled complexity: Why complex interventions are just not complicated enough. *Journal of Health Services Research & Policy* 2013;**18**(1):40–43.

37. Marchal B, Westhorp G, Wong G, et al. Realist RCTs of complex interventions: An oxymoron. *Social Science and Medicine* 2013;**94**:124–28.

38. Van Belle S, Wong G, Westhorp G, et al. Can 'realist' randomised controlled trials be genuinely realist? *Trials* 2016;**17**:313.

39. Craig P, Dieppe P, Macintyre S, et al. Developing and evaluating complex interventions: The new Medical Research Council guidance. *British Medical Journal* 2008;**337**:a1655.

40. Weinberger M, Oddone EZ, Henderson WG, et al. Multisite randomized controlled trials in health services research: Scientific challenges and operational issues. *Medical Care* 2001;**39**(6):627–34.

41. Banerjee AV, Duflo E. The experimental approach to development economics. *Annual Review of Economics* 2009;**1**:151–78.

42. Torgerson CJ, Torgerson DJ, Birks YF, et al. A comparison of randomised

controlled trials in health and education. *British Educational Research Journal* 2005;**31**:761–85.

43. Bonell CP, Bennett R, Oakley AO. Sexual health should be subject to experimental evaluation. In: Stephenson J, Imrie J, Bonell C, eds. *Effective Sexual Health Interventions: Issues in Experimental Evaluation*. Oxford: Oxford University Press 2003:3–16.

44. Chalmers I, Altman DG, eds. *Systematic Reviews*. London: BMJ Publishing Group 1995.

45. Littell JH, Corcoran J, Pillai V. *Systematic Reviews and Meta-Analysis*. Oxford: Oxford University Press 2008.

46. Brewin CR, Bradley C. Patient preferences and randomised controlled trials. *British Medical Journal* 1989;**299**:313–15.

47. Bonell C, Hargreaves JR, Strange V, et al. Should structural interventions be evaluated using RCTs? The case of HIV prevention. *Social Science & Medicine* 2007;**63**(5):1135–42.

48. Grijalva CG, Nuorti JP, Arbogast PJ, et al. Decline in pneumonia admissions after routine childhood immunisation with pneumococcal conjugate vaccine in the USA: A time-series analysis. *Lancet* 2007;**369**:1179–86.

49. Armstrong Schellenberg JR, Adam T, Mshinda H, et al. Effectiveness and cost of facility-based Integrated Management of Childhood Illness (IMCI) in Tanzania. *Lancet* 2004;**364**(9445):1583–94.

50. Cowan F, Plummer M. Biological, behavioural and psychological outcome measures. In: Stephenson J, Imrie J, Bonell C, eds. *Effective Sexual Health Interventions: Issues in Experimental Evaluation*. Oxford: Oxford University Press 2003:111–35.

51. Ogilvie D, Foster CE, Rothnie H, et al. Interventions to promote walking: Systematic review. *British Medical Journal* 2007;**334**:1204.

52. Criado Perez C. *Invisible Women: Exposing Data Bias in a World Designed for Men*. London: Random House 2019.

53. Gardner F, Montgomery P, Knerr W. Transporting evidence-based parenting programs for child problem behavior (age 3–10) between countries: Systematic review and meta-analysis. *Journal of Clinical Child & Adolescent Psychology* 2016;**45**(6):749–62.

54. Baker M. 1,500 scientists lift the lid on reproducibility. *Nature* 2016;**533**(7604):452–4.

55. Burchett HED, Kneale D, Blanchard L, et al. When assessing generalisability, focusing on differences in population or setting alone is insufficient. *Trials* 2020;**21**(1):286. https://doi.org/10.1186/s13063-020-4178-6.

56. Kelly JA, St Lawrence JA, Stevenson LY, et al. Community AIDS/HIV risk reduction: The effects of endorsements by popular people in three cities. *American Journal of Public Health* 1992;**82**(11):1483–89.

57. Williamson LM, Hart GJ, Flowers P, et al. The Gay Men's Task Force: The impact of peer education on the sexual health behaviour of homosexual men in Glasgow. *Sexually Transmitted Infections* 2001;**77**:427–32.

58. Kelly JA. Popular opinion leaders and HIV prevention peer education: Resolving discrepant findings, and implications for the development of effective community programmes. *AIDS Care* 2004;**16**(2):139–50.

59. Hart GJ, Williamson LM, Flowers P. Good in parts: The Gay Men's Task Force in Glasgow – a response to Kelly. *AIDS Care* 2004;**16**(2):159–65.

60. Pawson R. *Evidence-Based Policy: A Realist Perspective*. Thousand Oaks, CA: SAGE 2006.

61. Pawson R, Tilley N. *Realistic Evaluation*. London: SAGE 1997.

62. Cartwright N, Hardie J. *Evidence-Based Policy: A Practical Guide to Doing It Better*. Oxford: Oxford University Press 2012.

63. Whitehead M. A typology of actions to tackle social inequalities in health. *Journal of Epidemiol and Community Health* 2007;**61**(6):473–78.

64. Bryan CJ, Tipton E, Yeager DS. Behavioural science is unlikely to change the world without a heterogeneity revolution. *Nature Human Behaviour* 2021;**5**:980–89.

65. Fagan AA, Mihalic S. Strategies for enhancing the adoption of school-based prevention programs: Lessons learned from the blueprints for violence prevention replications of the life skills training program. *Journal of Community Psychology* 2003;**31**(3):235–53.

66. Glasgow RE, Vogt TM, Boles SM. Evaluating the public health impact of health promotion interventions: The RE-AIM framework. *American Journal of Public Health* 1999;**89**:1322–27.

67. Petticrew M. Time to rethink the systematic review catechism? Moving from 'what works' to 'what happens'. *Systematic Reviews* 2015;**4**(1):36.

68. Oakley A, Strange V, Bonell C, et al. Integrating process evaluation in the design of randomised controlled trials of complex interventions: The example of the RIPPLE study. *British Medical Journal* 2006;**332**:413–16.

69. Strange V, Forrest S, Oakley A, et al. Peer-led sex education–characteristics of peer educators and their perceptions of the impact on them of participation in a peer education programme. *Health Education Research* 2002;**17**(3):327–37.

70. Coker AL, Bush HM, Brancato CJ, et al. Bystander program effectiveness to reduce violence acceptance: RCT in high schools. *Journal of Family Violence* 2019;**34**(3):153–64.

71. Main C, Thomas S, Ogilvie D, et al. Population tobacco control interventions and their effects on social inequalities in smoking: Placing an equity lens on existing systematic reviews. *BMC Public Health* 2008;**8**:178.

72. Farrington DP, Ttofi MM. School-based programs to reduce bullying and victimization. *Campbell Systematic Reviews* 2009;**5**(1):1–148.

73. Lipsey MW. The primary factors that characterize effective interventions with juvenile offenders: A meta-analytic overview. *Victims and Offenders* 2009;**4**:124–47.

74. Bhaskar R. *A Realist Theory of Science*. Leeds: Leeds Books 1975.

75. Bhaskar R. *The Possibility of Naturalism: A Philosophical Critique of the Contemporary Human Sciences*. Brighton: Harvester 1979.

76. Sherman L. *Policing Domestic Violence*. New York: Free Press 1992.

77. Dalkin SM, Greenhalgh J, Jones D, et al. What's in a mechanism? Development of a key concept in realist evaluation. *Implementation Science* 2015;**10**(1):1–7.

78. Blackwood B, O'Halloran P, Porter S. On the problems of mixing RCTs with qualitative research: The case of the MRC framework for the evaluation of complex healthcare interventions. *Journal of Research in Nursing* 2010;**15**(6):511–21.

79. Hawkins AJ. Realist evaluation and randomised controlled trials for testing program theory in complex social systems. *Evaluation* 2016;**22**(3):270–85.

80. Blaikie N. *Approaches to Social Enquiry*. Cambridge: Polity Press 1993.

81. Comte A. *The Positive Philosophy of Auguste Comte*. Cambridge: Cambridge University Press 2010.

82. Godfrey-Smith P. *Theory and Reality: An Introduction to the Philosophy of Science*. Chicago: University of Chicago Press 2010.

83. Wong G, Greenhalgh T, Westhorp G, et al. RAMESES publication standards: Realist syntheses. *BMC Medicine* 2013;**11**:21.

84. Pawson R, Greenhalgh T, Harvey G, et al. Realist review – a new method of systematic review designed for complex policy interventions. *Journal of Health Services Research & Policy* 2005;**10**:21–34.

85. Rose G. *The Strategy of Preventive Medicine*. Oxford: Oxford University Press 1992.

86. Campbell R, Starkey F, Holliday J, et al. An informal school-based peer-led intervention for smoking prevention in adolescence (ASSIST): A cluster

randomised trial. *Lancet* 2008;**371**:1595–602.

87. Oakley A. *Experiments in Knowing: Gender and Method in the Social Sciences.* Cambridge: Polity Press 2000.

88. Habicht JP, Victora CG, Vaughan JP. Evaluation designs for adequacy, plausibility and probability of public health programme performance and impact. *International Journal of Epidemiology* 1999;**28**:10–18.

89. Schreuders M, Nuyts PAW, van den Putte B, et al. Understanding the impact of school tobacco policies on adolescent smoking behaviour: A realist review. *Social Science & Medicine* 2017;**183**(19):e27.

90. Defever E, Jones M. Rapid realist review of school-based physical activity interventions in 7- to 11–year-old children. *Children and Youth Services Review* 2021;**8**:52. https://doi.org/10.3390/children8010052.

91. Berg RC, Nanavati J. Realist review: Current practice and future prospects. *Journal of Research Practice* 2016;**12**:R1. http://jrp.icaap.org/index.php/jrp/article/view/538/449.

92. Bonell C, Moore G, Warren E, et al. Are randomized controlled trials positivist? Reviewing the social science and philosophy literature to assess positivist tendencies of trials of social interventions in public health and health services. *Trials* 2018;**19**:238.

93. Green J, Thorogood N. *Qualitative Methods for Health Research.* London: SAGE 2004.

94. Moore GF, Audrey S, Barker M, et al. Process evaluation of complex interventions: Medical Research Council guidance. *British Medical Journal* 2015;**350**:h1258.

95. Markham WA, Aveyard P. A new theory of health promoting schools based on human functioning, school organisation and pedagogic practice. *Social Science & Medicine* 2003;**56**(6):1209–20.

96. Bernstein B. *Class, Codes and Control, Vol. 3: Towards a Theory of Educational Transmission.* London: Routledge 1975.

97. Moher D, Hopewell S, Schulz KF, et al. CONSORT 2010 explanation and elaboration: Updated guidelines for reporting parallel group randomised trials. *British Medical Journal* 2010;**340**: c869.

98. Olds DL, Robinson J, O'Brien R, et al. Home visiting by paraprofessionals and by nurses: A randomized, controlled trial. *Pediatrics* 2002;**110**(3):486–96.

99. Robling M, Bekkers MJ, Bell K, et al. Effectiveness of a nurse-led intensive home-visitation programme for first-time teenage mothers (building blocks): A pragmatic randomised controlled trial. *Lancet* 2016;**387**(10014):146–55.

100. Langford R, Bonell CP, Jones HE, et al. The WHO Health Promoting School framework for improving the health and well-being of students and staff. *Cochrane Database of Systematic Reviews* 2014; Issue 1 Art No: CD008958.

101. Flay BR, Graumlich S, Segawa E, et al. Effects of 2 prevention programs on high-risk behaviors among African American youth: A randomized trial. *Archives Pediatrics and Adolescent Medicine* 2004;**158**(4):377–84. https://doi.org/10.1001/archpedi.158.4.377.

102. Weber M. *The Methodology of the Social Sciences.* Glencoe, IL: Free Press 1949.

103. May C. Towards a general theory of implementation. *Implementation Science* 2013;**8**:18.

104. Nilsen P. Making sense of implementation theories, models and frameworks. *Implementation Science* 2015;**10**:53.

105. Morgan DL. Practical strategies for combining qualitative and quantitative methods: Applications to health research. *Qualitative Health Research* 1998;**8**(3):362–76.

106. Weiss C. Nothing as practical as good theory: Exploring theory-based evaluation for comprehensive community initiatives for children and families. In: Connell JP, ed. *New Approaches to Evaluating Community Initiatives Concepts, Methods, and Contexts*

Roundtable on Comprehensive Community Initiatives for Children and Families. Washington, DC: Aspen Institute 1995:65–92.

107. Glanz K, Bishop D. The role of behavioral science theory in development and implementation of public health interventions. *Annual Review of Public Health* 2010;**31**:399–418.

108. Noar SM, Chabot M, Zimmerman RS. Applying health behavior theory to multiple behavior change: Considerations and approaches. *Preventive Medicine* 2008;**46**(3):275–80.

109. Breuer E, Lee L, De Silva M, et al. Using theory of change to design and evaluate public health interventions: A systematic review. *Implementation Science* 2016;**11**(1):63. https://doi.org/10.1186/s13012-016-0422-6.

110. Moore GF, Evans RE. What theory, for whom and in which context? Reflections on the application of theory in the development and evaluation of complex population health interventions. *Social Science and Medicine Population Health* 2017;**3**:132–35.

111. Lemire S, Kwako AJ, Nielsen SB, et al. What is this thing called a mechanism? Findings from a review of published realist evaluations. *New Directions for Evaluation* 2020;**167**:73–86.

112. Connell JP, Kubisch AC. *Applying a Theory of Change Approach to the Evaluation of Comprehensive Community Initiatives: Progress, Prospects, and Problems.* Washington, DC: The Aspen Institute 1998.

113. Patton MQ. *Qualitative Research & Evaluation Methods* (3rd ed.). Thousand Oaks, CA: SAGE 2002.

114. Walton GM, Yeager DS. Seed and soil: Psychological affordances in contexts help to explain where wise interventions succeed or fail. *Current Directions in Psychological Science* 2020;**29**(3):219–26.

115. Carey RN, Connell LE, Johnston M, et al. Behavior change techniques and their mechanisms of action: A synthesis of links described in published intervention literature. *Annals of Behavioral Medicine* 2019;**53**(8):693–707.

116. Giddens A. *The Constitution of Society.* Cambridge: Polity Press 1984.

117. Marchal B, van Belle S, van Olmen J, et al. Is realist evaluation keeping its promise? A review of published empirical studies in the field of health systems. *Evaluation* 2012;**18**(2):192–212.

118. Falleti TG, Lynch JF. Context and causal mechanisms in political analysis. *Comparative Political Studies* 2009;**42**(9):1143–66.

119. Hedstrom P, Swedberg R. *Social Mechanisms: An Analytical Approach to Social Theory.* Cambridge: Cambridge University Press 1998.

120. Astbury B, Leeuw FL. Unpacking black boxes: Mechanisms and theory building in evaluation. *American Journal of Evaluation* 2010;**31**(3):363–81.

121. Sayer A. *Realism and Social Science.* London: SAGE 2000.

122. Jansen YJFM, Foets MME, de Bont AA. The contribution of qualitative research to the development of tailor-made community-based interventions in primary care: A review. *European Journal of Public Health* 2010;**20**(2):220–26.

123. Barnes M, Matka E, Sullivan H. Evidence, understanding and complexity: Evaluation in non-linear systems. *Evaluation* 2003;**9**:265–84.

124. Porter S. The uncritical realism of realist evaluation. *Evaluation* 2015;**21**(1):65–82.

125. Bonell C, Allen E, Warren E, et al. Initiating change in the school environment to reduce bullying and aggression: A cluster randomised controlled trial of the Learning Together (LT) intervention in English secondary schools. *Lancet* 2018;**392**(10163):2452–64.

126. Jamal F, Fletcher A, Shackleton A, et al. The three stages of building and testing mid-level theories in a realist RCT: A case-example. *Trials* 2015;**16**:466.

127. Campbell R, Bonell C. Development and evaluation of complex interventions in

public health. In: Detels R, Beaglehole MA, Lansang M, et al., eds. *Oxford Textbook of Public Health*, 7th ed. Oxford: Oxford University Press 2014:751–60.

128. van Urk F, Grant S, Bonell C. Involving stakeholders in programme theory specification: Discussion of a systematic, consensus-based approach. *Evidence & Policy* 2016;**12**(14):541–57.

129. Nussbaum MC. Aristotelian social democracy. In: Douglas RB, Mara GM, Richardson H, eds. *Liberalism and the Good*. London: Routledge 1990:203–51.

130. Tobler AL, Komro KA, Dabroski A, et al. Preventing the link between SES and high-risk behaviors: 'Value-added' education, drug use and delinquency in high-risk, urban schools. *Prevention Science* 2011;**12**(2):211–21.

131. Markham WA, Aveyard P, Bisset SL, et al. Value-added education and smoking uptake in schools: A cohort study. *Addiction* 2008;**103**(1):155–61.

132. Bonell CP, Parry W, Wells H, et al. The effects of the school environment on student health: A systematic review of multi-level studies. *Health and Place* 2013;**21**:180–91.

133. Bonell C, Sorhaindo A, Allen E, et al. Pilot multi-method trial of a school-ethos intervention to reduce substance use: Building hypotheses about upstream pathways to prevention. *Journal of Adolescent Health* 2010;**47**(6):555–63.

134. Bond L, Glover S, Godfrey C, et al. Building capacity for system-level change in schools: Lessons from the Gatehouse project. *Health Education and Behavior* 2001;**28**(3):368–83.

135. Fletcher A, Jamal F, Moore G, et al. Realist complex intervention science: Applying realist principles across all phases of the Medical Research Council framework for developing and evaluating complex interventions. *Evaluation* 2016;**22**(3):286–303.

136. Pearson M, Chilton R, Wyatt K, et al. Implementing health promotion programmes in schools: A realist systematic review of research and experience in the United Kingdom. *Implementation Science* 2015;**10**(1):1.

137. Jamal F, Fletcher A, Harden A, et al. The school environment and student health: A systematic review and meta-ethnography of qualitative research. *BMC Public Health* 2013;**13**(1):798.

138. Popper K. *The Open Society and Its Enemies*, Volume 2 Hegel and Marx. London: Routledge 1945.

139. Buckley S, Maxwell GM. *Respectful Schools: Restorative Practices in Education: A Summary Report*. Wellington: Office of the Children's Commissioner and the Institute of Policy Studies, School of Government. Victoria, Australia: Victoria University 2007.

140. Garandeau CF, Salmivalli C. Can healthier contexts be harmful? A new perspective on the plight of victims of bullying. *Child Development Perspectives* 2019;**13**(3):147–52.

141. Unrau YA. Using client exit interviews to illuminate outcomes in program logic models: A case example. *Evaluation and Program Planning* 2001;**24**:353–61.

142. Glaser D. Child abuse and neglect and the brain–a review. *Journal of Child Psychology and Psychiatry* 2000;**41**(1):97–116.

143. Steckler L, Linnan A, eds. *Process Evaluation for Public Health Interventions and Research*. San Francisco: Jossey-Bass 2004.

144. Michie S, Van Stralen MM, West R. The behaviour change wheel: A new method for characterising and designing behaviour change interventions. *Implementation Science* 2011;**6**(1):42.

145. Hoffmann TC, Glasziou PP, Boutron I, et al. Better reporting of interventions: Template for intervention description and replication (TIDieR) checklist and guide. *British Medical Journal* 2014;**348**: g1687.

146. Bonell C, Fletcher A, Fitzgerald-Yau N, et al. A pilot randomised controlled trial

of the INCLUSIVE intervention for initiating change locally in bullying and aggression through the school environment: Final report. *Health Technology Assessment* 2015;**19**(53):1–109.

147. Bonell C, Allen E, Warren E, et al. Initiating change locally in bullying and aggression through the school environment: The INCLUSIVE cluster RCT. *Public Health Research* 2019;**7**(18):1–196.

148. Warren E, Opondo C, Allen E, et al. Action groups as a participative strategy for leading whole-school health promotion: Results on implementation from the INCLUSIVE trial in English secondary schools. *British Education Research Journal* 2019;**45**(5):748–62.

149. Warren E, Melendez-Torres GJ, Viner RM, et al. Using qualitative research within a realist trial to build theory about how context and mechanisms interact to generate outcomes: Findings from the INCLUSIVE trial of a whole-school health intervention. *Trials* 2020;**21**:774.

150. Pawson R. Theorizing the interview. *British Journal of Sociology* 1996;**47**(2):295–314.

151. Manzano A. The craft of interviewing in realist evaluation. *Evaluation* 2016;**22**(3):342–60.

152. Schatzman L. Dimensional analysis: Notes on an alternative approach to the grounding of theory in qualitative research. In: Maines D, ed. *Social Organization and Social Process: Essays in Honor of Anselm Strauss*. New York: Aldine 1991:303–14.

153. Thirsk LM, Clark AM. Using qualitative research for complex interventions: The contributions of hermeneutics. *International Journal of Qualitative Methods* 2017;**16**:1–10.

154. Charmaz K. *Constructing Grounded Theory*. New York: SAGE 2014.

155. Blumer H. *Symbolic Interactionism: Perspective and Method*. Englewood Cliffs, NJ: Prentice Hall 1969.

156. Oliver C. Critical realist grounded theory: A new approach for social work research. *British Journal of Social Work* 2011;**42**(2):371–87.

157. Hoddy E. Critical realism in empirical research: Employing techniques from grounded theory methodology. *International Journal of Social Research Methodology* 2018;**22**:111–24.

158. Munro A, Bloor M. Process evaluation: The new miracle ingredient in public health research? *Qualitative Research* 2010;**10**(6):699–713.

159. Lancaster GA. Pilot and feasibility studies come of age! *Pilot and Feasibility Studies* 2015;**1**(1):1–1.

160. Campbell M, Fitzpatrick R, Haines A, et al. Framework for design and evaluation of complex interventions to improve health. *British Medical Journal* 2000;**321**:694–96.

161. Bonell CP, Fletcher A, Fitzgerald-Yau N, et al. Initiating change locally in bullying and aggression through the school environment (INCLUSIVE): Pilot randomised controlled trial. *Health Technology Assessment* 2015;**19**(53):1–110.

162. Audrey S, Holliday J, Parry-Langdon N, et al. Meeting the challenges of implementing process evaluation within randomized controlled trials: The example of ASSIST (A Stop Smoking in Schools Trial). *Health Education Research* 2006;**21**(3):366–77.

163. Wilkinson R, Pickett K. *The Spirit Level: Why More Equal Societies Almost Always Do Better*. London: Allen Lane 2009.

164. Marmot MG. *Fair Society, Healthy Lives: The Marmot Review. Strategic Review of Health Inequalities in England post-2010*. London: The Marmot Review 2010.

165. Bonell C, Fletcher A, Morton M, et al. 'Realist randomised controlled trials': A new approach to evaluating complex

public health interventions. *Social Science and Medicine* 2012;75(12):2299–306.

166. Warren E, Melendez-Torres GJ, Bonell C. Are realist randomised controlled trials possible? A reflection on the INCLUSIVE evaluation of a whole-school, bullying-prevention intervention. *Trials* 2022;23(82). https://doi.org/10.1186/s130 63-021-05976-1.

167. Tipton E, Yeager DS, Iachan R, et al. *Designing Probability Samples to Identify Sources of Treatment Effect Heterogeneity.* New York: Wiley 2019:435–56.

168. Patton G, Bond L, Carlin JB, et al. Promoting social inclusion in schools: Group-randomized trial of effects on student health risk behaviour and well-being. *American Journal of Public Health* 2006;96(9):1582–87.

169. Petticrew M, Tugwell P, Kristjannsson E, et al. Damned if you do, damned if you don't: Subgroup analysis and equity. *Journal of Epidemiology and Community Health* 2012;66:95–98.

170. Torgerson D, Sibbald B. Understanding controlled trials: What is a patient preference trial? *British Medical Journal* 1998;316:360.

171. Hussey MA, Hughes JP. Design and analysis of stepped wedge cluster randomized trials. *Contemporary Clinical Trials* 2007;28:182–91.

172. Bonell C, Hargreaves J, Cousens S, et al. Alternatives to randomisation in the evaluation of public-health interventions: Design challenges and solutions. *Journal of Epidemiology and Community Health* 2011;65(7):582–87.

173. Cousens S, Hargreaves J, Bonell C, et al. Alternatives to randomisation in the evaluation of public-health interventions: Statistical analysis and causal inference. *Journal of Epidemiology and Community Health* 2011;65(7):576–81.

174. Egan M, Petticrew M, Ogilvie D, et al. New roads and human health: A systematic review. *American Journal of Public Health* 2003;93(9):1463–71.

175. Hutchinson P, Wheeler J. Advanced methods for evaluating the impact of family planning communication programs: Evidence from Tanzania and Nepal. *Studies in Family Planning* 2006;37(3):169–86.

176. Bonell C, Dodd M, Allen E, et al. Broader impacts of an intervention to transform school environments on student behaviour and school functioning: Post hoc analyses from the INCLUSIVE cluster randomised controlled trial. *BMJ Open* 2020;10(5):e031589.

177. Wigelsworth M, Thornton E, Troncoso P, et al. *A Whole-School Approach to Improving Behaviour and Reducing Bullying: An Independent Evaluation of the 'INCLUSIVE' Project.* London: Education Endowment Foundation 2023.

178. Williams J, Miller S, Cutbush S, et al. A latent transition model of the effects of a teen dating violence prevention initiative. *Journal of Adolescent Health* 2015;56:eS32.

179. Melendez-Torres GJ, Allen E, Viner R, et al. Effects of a whole-school health intervention on clustered adolescent health risks: Latent transition analysis of data from the INCLUSIVE trial. *Prevention Science* 2022;23(1):1–9.

180. Frazier PA, Tix AP, Barron KE. Testing moderator and mediator effects in counseling psychology research. *Journal of Counseling and Psychology* 2013;67(2):190–3.

181. Lorenc T, Petticrew M, Welch V, et al. What types of interventions generate inequalities? Evidence from systematic reviews. *Journal of Epidemiology and Community Health Online First* 2012. http://jechbmjcom/content/early/2012/08 /07/jech-2012-201257full.

182. Murphy SM, Edwards RT, Williams N, et al. An evaluation of the effectiveness and cost effectiveness of the National Exercise Referral Scheme in Wales, UK: A randomised controlled trial of a public health policy initiative. *Journal of Epidemiology and Community Health* 2012;66(8):745–53.

183. Turnwald BP, Bertoldo JD, Perry MA, et al. Increasing vegetable intake by emphasizing tasty and enjoyable attributes: A randomized controlled multisite intervention for taste-focused labeling. *Psychology Science* 2019;**30**(11):1603–15.

184. Shackleton N, Fletcher A, Jamal F, et al. A new measure of unhealthy school environments and its implications for critical assessments of health promotion in schools. *Critical Public Health* 2017;**27**(2):248–62.

185. Sawyer MG, Pfeiffer S, Spence SH, et al. School-based prevention of depression: A randomised controlled study of the beyond blue schools research initiative. *Journal of Child Psychology and Psychiatry* 2010;**51**(2):199–209.

186. Baron RM, Kenny DA. The moderator-mediator variable distinction in social psychological research: Conceptual, strategic and statistical considerations. *Journal of Personality and Social Psychology* 1986;**51**:1173–82.

187. MacKinnon DP, Lockwood CM, Hoffman JM, et al. A comparison of methods to test mediation and other intervening variable effects. *Psychological Methods* 2002;**7**:83–104.

188. Bonell C, Allen E, Opondo C, et al. Examining intervention mechanisms of action using mediation analysis within a randomised trial of a whole-school health intervention. *Journal of Epidemiology and Community Health* 2019;**73**(5):455–64.

189. Littlecott HJ, Moore G, Moore L, et al. Psychosocial mediators of change in physical activity in the Welsh national exercise referral scheme: Secondary analysis of a randomised controlled trial. *International Journal of Behavior, Nutrition and Physical Activity* 2014;**11**:109.

190. Melendez-Torres GJ, Warren E, Viner R, et al. Moderated mediation analyses to assess intervention mechanisms for impacts on victimisation, psycho-social problems and mental wellbeing: Evidence from the INCLUSIVE realist randomized

trial. *Social Science and Medicine* 2021;**279**:113984.

191. Melendez-Torres GJ, Warren E, Ukoumunne O, et al. Locating and testing the healthy context paradox: Examples from the INCLUSIVE trial. *BMC Medical Research Methodology* 2022;**22**(1):57. https://doi.org/10.1186/s12874-022-01537-5.

192. Ragin CC. Turning the tables: How case-oriented research challenges. *Rethinking Social Inquiry: Diverse Tools, Shared Standards* 2004;123–38.

193. Ragin CC. *Redesigning Social Inquiry: Fuzzy Sets and Beyond*. Chicago: University of Chicago Press 2009.

194. Ragin CC, Becker HS. What Is a Case? Exploring the Foundations of Social Inquiry. Cambridge: Cambridge University Press 1992.

195. Rihoux B, Ragin CC. *Configurational Comparative Methods: Qualitative Comparative Analysis (QCA) and Related Techniques*. New York: SAGE 2008.

196. Thomas J, O'Mara-Eves A, Brunton G. Using Qualitative Comparative Analysis (QCA) in systematic reviews of complex interventions: A worked example. *Systematic Reviews* 2014;**3**(1):67.

197. Warren E, Melendez-Torres GJ, Bonell C. Using fuzzy-set qualitative comparative analysis to explore causal pathways to reduced bullying in a whole-school intervention in a randomized controlled trial. *Journal of School Violence* 2022;**21**(4):381–96.

198. Sager F, Andereggen C. Dealing with complex causality in realist synthesis: The promise of qualitative comparative analysis. *American Journal of Evaluation* 2012;**33**(1):60–78.

199. Bonell C, Prost A, Melendez-Torres G, et al. Will it work here? A realist approach to local decisions about implementing interventions evaluated as effective elsewhere. *Journal of Epidemiology and Community Health* 2021;**75**(1):46–50.

200. Pawson R. *The Science of Evaluation: A Realist Manifesto*. London: SAGE 2013.

201. Catalano RF, Berglund LM, Ryan JAM, et al. Positive youth development in the United States: Research findings on evaluations of positive youth development programs. *Prevention & Treatment* 2002;5(1):1–166.

202. Harden A, Brunton G, Fletcher A, et al. Teenage pregnancy and social disadvantage: A systematic review integrating trials and qualitative studies. *British Medical Journal* 2009;339:b4254.

203. Kirby D. *Emerging Answers: Research Findings on Programs to Reduce Teen Pregnancy.* Washington, DC: National Campaign to Prevent Teen Pregnancy 2001.

204. Armstrong R, Waters E, Moore L, et al. Improving the reporting of public health intervention research: Advancing TREND and CONSORT. *Journal of Public Health* 2008;30(1):103–09.

205. Loxton D, Dolja-Gore X, Anderson AE, et al. Intimate partner violence adversely impacts health over 16 years and across generations: A longitudinal cohort study. *PLoS One* 2017;12(6):e0178138. https://doi.org/10.1371/journal.pone.0178138.

206. Costa BM, Kaestle CE, Walker A, et al. Longitudinal predictors of domestic violence perpetration and victimization: A systematic review. *Aggressive and Violent Behaviour* 2015;24:261–72.

207. Fellmeth GLT, Heffernan C, Nurse J, et al. Educational and skills-based interventions for preventing relationship and dating violence in adolescents and young adults: Cochrane database. *Systematic Reviews* 2013;Art No. CD004534. https://doi.org/10.1002/14651858.CD004534.

208. De La Rue L, Polanin JR, Espelage DL, et al. A meta-analysis of school-based interventions aimed to prevent or reduce violence in teen dating relationships. *Review of Educational Research* 2016;87(1):7–34.

209. Kettrey HH, Marx RA, Tanner-Smith EE. Effects of bystander programs on the prevention of sexual assault among adolescents and college students: A systematic review. *Campbell Systematic Reviews* 2019;15:e1013.

210. Stanley N, Ellis J, Farrelly N, et al. Preventing domestic abuse for children and young people: A review of school-based interventions. *Children and Youth Services Review* 2015;59:120–31.

211. Lundgren R, Amin A. Addressing intimate partner violence and sexual violence among adolescents: Emerging evidence of effectiveness. *Journal of Adolescent Health* 2015;56:S42–50.

212. Munoz-Fernandez N, Ortega-Rivera J, Nocentini A, et al. The efficacy of the 'Dat-E adolescence' prevention program in the reduction of dating violence and bullying. *International Journal of Environmental Research and Public Health* 2019;16(3):408. https://doi.org/10.3390/ijerph16030408.

213. Gage AJ, Honoré JG, Deleon J. *Pilot Test of a Dating Violence-Prevention Curriculum among High School Students: Emerging Evidence of Effectiveness in a Low-Income Country.* 2016. Measure Evaluation. See www.measureevaluation.org/publications/wp-14-149.html.

214. Devries KM, Knight L, Allen E, et al. Does the good schools toolkit reduce physical, sexual and emotional violence, and injuries, in girls and boys equally? A cluster-randomised controlled trial. *Prevention Science* 2017;18(7):839–53. https://doi.org/10.1007/s11121-017-0775-3.

215. Noblit G, Hare R. *Meta-Ethnography: Synthesizing Qualitative Studies.* London: SAGE 1988.

216. Orr N, Chollet A, Rizzo A, et al. School-based interventions for preventing dating and relationship violence and gender-based violence: A systematic review and synthesis of theories of change. *Review of Educational Research* 2022;10(3):e3382.

217. Shepherd J, Kavanagh J, Picot J, et al. The effectiveness and cost-effectiveness of behavioural interventions for the prevention of sexually transmitted infections in young people aged 13 to 19: A systematic review and economic

evaluation. *Health Technology Assessment Monographs* 2010;**14**(7):1–206.

218. Herlitz L, MacIntyre H, Osborn T, et al. The sustainability of public health interventions in schools: A systematic review. *Implementation Science* 2020;**15**(1):4.

219. Tancred T, Paparini S, Melendez-Torres GJ, et al. Interventions integrating health and academic interventions to prevent substance use and violence: A systematic review and synthesis of process evaluations. *Systematic Reviews* 2018;**7**:227.

220. Bonell C, Dickson K, Hinds K, et al. The effects of Positive Youth Development interventions on substance use, violence and inequalities: Systematic review of theories of change, processes and outcomes. *Public Health Research* 2016;**4**(5):1–218.

221. Bonell C, Jamal F, Harden A, et al. Systematic review of the effects of schools and school environment interventions on health: Evidence mapping and synthesis. *Public Health Research* 2013;**1**(1):1–320.

222. Tancred T, Melendez-Torres GJ, Paparini S, et al. Interventions integrating health and academic education in schools to prevent substance misuse and violence: Systematic review and evidence synthesis. *Public Health Research* 2018;**7**(17):1–244.

223. Ponsford R, Melendez-Torres GJ, Miners A, et al. Whole-school interventions promoting student commitment to school to prevent substance use and violence and improve educational attainment: A systematic review. *Public Health Research* 2023;**221**:190–197.

224. Meiksin R, Melendez-Torres GJ, Miners A, et al. E-health interventions targeting HIV/STIs, sexual risk, substance use and mental ill-health among men who have sex with men: Systematic review. *Public Health Research* 2022;**10**(4):1–352.

225. Farmer C, Shaw N, Rizzo AJ, et al. School-based interventions to prevent dating and relationship violence and gender-based violence: Systematic review and network meta-analysis. *American Journal of Public Health* 2023;**113**(3):320–30.

226. Wekerle C, Waechter RL, Leung E, et al. Adolescence: A window of opportunity for positive change in mental health. *First Peoples Child & Family Review* 2007;**3**(2):8–16.

227. Jewkes R, Flood M, Lang J. From work with men and boys to changes of social norms and reduction of inequities in gender relations: A conceptual shift in prevention of violence against women and girls. *Lancet* 2014;**104**(1):F8–F12. https://doi.org/101016/S0140-6736(14)61683-4.

228. Dias S, Caldwell DMA. Network meta-analysis explained. *Archives of Disease in Childhood Fetal and Neonatal Edition* 2019;**104**:F8–12.

229. Espelage DL, Low S, Polanin JR, et al. The impact of a middle school program to reduce aggression, victimization, and sexual violence. *Journal of Adolescent Health* 2013;**53**(2):180–6. https://doi.org/10.1016/j.jadohealth.2013.02.021.

230. Thompson SG. Why sources of heterogeneity in meta-analysis should be investigated. *British Medical Journal* 1994;**309**:1351–55.

231. Greenland S, Robins J. Ecologic studies-biases, misconceptions, and counterexamples. *American Journal of Epidemiology* 1994;**139**:747–60.

232. Thomas J, O'Mara-Eves A, Brunton G. Using Qualitative Comparative Analysis (QCA) in systematic reviews of complex interventions: A worked example. *Systematic Reviews* 2014;**3**:67.

233. Melendez-Torres G, Sutcliffe K, Burchett HE, et al. Developing and testing intervention theory by incorporating a views synthesis into a qualitative comparative analysis of intervention effectiveness. *Research Synthesis Methods* 2019;**10**(3):389–97.

234. Kneale D, Rojas-García A, Thomas J. Obstacles and opportunities to using research evidence in local public health decision-making in England. *Health Research Policy and Systems* 2019;**17**:61.

235. Loren T, Oliver K. Adverse effects of public health interventions: A conceptual framework. *Journal of Epidemiology and Community Health* 2014;**68**(3):288–90.

236. Kirke DM. Chain reactions in adolescents' cigarette, alcohol and drug use: Similarity through peer influence or the patterning of ties in peer networks? *Social Networks* 2004;**26**:3–28.

237. Freedman B. Equipoise and the ethics of clinical research. *New England Journal of Medicine* 1987;**317**:141–45.

238. Bonell C, Prost A, Melendez-Torres GJ, et al. Will it work here? A realist approach to local decisions about implementing interventions evaluated as effective elsewhere. *Journal of Epidemiology and Community Health* 2021;**75**(1):46–50.

239. Evans R, Murphy S, Scourfield J. Implementation of a school-based social and emotional learning intervention: Understanding diffusion processes within complex systems. *Prevention Science* 2015;**16**(5):754–64.

240. Romasz TE, Kantor JH, Elias MJ. Implementation and evaluation of urban school-wide social–emotional learning programs. *Evaluation and Program Planning* 2004;**27**(1):89–103.

241. Movsisyan A, Arnold L, Evans R, et al. Adapting evidence-informed complex population health interventions for new contexts: A systematic review of guidance. *Implementation Science* 2019;**14**(1):105.

242. Munthe-Kaas H, Nøkleby H, Lewin S, et al. The TRANSFER approach for assessing the transferability of systematic review findings. *BMC Medical Research Methodology* 2020;**20**(1):11.

243. Lewis KM, Bavarian N, Snyder FJ, et al. Direct and mediated effects of a social-emotional and character development program on adolescent substance use. *International Journal of Emotional Education* 2012;**4**(1):1–14.

244. Durlak JA, Weissberg RP, Dymnicki AB. The impact of enhancing students' social and emotional learning: A meta-analysis of school-based universal interventions. *Child Development* 2011;**82**(1):405–32.

245. Goldberg JM, Sklad M, Elfrink TR, et al. Effectiveness of interventions adopting a whole school approach to enhancing social and emotional development: A meta-analysis. *European Journal of Psychology of Education* 2019;**34**:755–82.

246. Blewitt C, Fuller-Tyszkiewicz M, Nolan A, et al. Social and emotional learning associated with universal curriculum-based interventions in early childhood education and care centers: A systematic review and meta-analysis. *JAMA Network Open* 2018;**1**(8):e185727.

247. Belfield C, Bowden B, Klapp A, et al. The economic value of social and emotional learning. New York: Center for Benefit-Cost Studies in Education, Teachers College, Columbia University 2015.

248. Corcoran RP, Cheung ACK, Kim E, et al. Effective universal school-based social and emotional learning programs for improving academic achievement: A systematic review and meta-analysis of 50 years of research. *Educational Research Review* 2018;**25**:56–72.

249. Escoffery C, Lebow-Skelley E, Udelson H, et al. A scoping study of frameworks for adapting public health evidence-based interventions. *Translational Behavioral Medicine* 2019;**9**(1):1–10.

250. Pfadenhauer LM, Gerhardus A, Mozygemba K, et al. Making sense of complexity in context and implementation: The Context and Implementation of Complex Interventions (CICI) framework. *Implementation Science* 2017;**12**:21.

251. Thomson KC, Richardson CG, Gadermann AM, et al. Association of childhood social-emotional functioning profiles at school entry with early-onset mental health conditions. *JAMA Network Open* 2019;**2**(1):e186694.

252. Korteweg HA, van Bokhoven I, Yzermans C, et al. Rapid health and needs assessments after disasters: A systematic review. *BMC Public Health* 2010;**10**:295.

253. Aarons GA, Sklar M, Mustanski B, et al. Scaling-out evidence-based interventions to new populations or new health care delivery systems. *Implementation Science* 2017;**12**(1):111.

254. Hargreaves J, Hatcher A, Strange V, et al. Process evaluation of the Intervention with Microfinance for AIDS and Gender Equity (IMAGE) in rural South Africa. *Health Education Research* 2009;**25**(1):27–40.

255. Durlak JA, DuPre EP. Implementation matters: A review of research on the influence of implementation on program outcomes and the factors affecting implementation. *American Journal of Community Psychology* 2008;**41**:327–50.

256. European Centre for Disease Prevention and Control. *The Use of Evidence in Decision-Making during Public Health Emergencies: Report on an Expert Workshop*. Stockholm: European Centre for Disease Prevention and Control 2019.

257. Warsame A, Blanchet K, Checchi F. Towards systematic evaluation of epidemic responses during humanitarian crises: A scoping review of existing public health evaluation frameworks. *BMJ Global Health* 2020;**5**:e002109.

258. Diderichsen F, Evans T, Whitehead M. The social basis of disparities in health. In: Evans T, Whitehead M, Diderichsen F, et al., eds. *Challenging Inequities in Health*. New York: Oxford University Press 2001:12–23.

259. Bonell C, Jamal F, Melendez-Torres GJ, et al. 'Dark logic' – theorising the harmful consequences of public health interventions. *Journal of Epidemiology and Community Health* 2015;**69**(1):95–8.

260. Matuchansky C. The promise of personalised medicine. *Lancet* 2015;**386**(9995):742.

261. National Institute for Health and Clinical Excellence. School-based interventions to prevent smoking (Quick reference guide). London: NICE 2010.

262. Bonell C, Ponsford R, Meiksin R, et al. Testing and refining middle-range theory in evaluations of public-health interventions: Evidence from recent systematic reviews and trials. *Journal of Epidemiology and Community Health* 2023;**77**(3):147–51.

263. Starkey F, Audrey S, Holliday J, et al. Identifying influential young people to undertake effective peer-led health promotion: The example of A Stop Smoking In Schools Trial (ASSIST). *Health Education Research* 2009;**24**(6):977–88.

264. Rogers EM. *Diffusion of Innovations*. New York: The Free Press 1962.

265. Lunn P, Belton C, Lavin C, et al. Using behavioural science to help fight the Coronavirus. Economic and Social Research Institute 2020. www.esri.ie/pub lications/using-behavioural-science-to-he lp-fight-the-coronavirus.

266. Bonell C, Michie S, Reicher S, et al. Harnessing behavioural science in public health campaigns to maintain 'social distancing' in response to the COVID-19 pandemic: Key principles. *Journal of Epidemiology and Community Health* 2020;**74**(8):617–19.

267. Drury J, Carter H, Cocking C, et al. Facilitating collective resilience in the public in emergencies: Twelve recommendations based on the social identity approach. *Frontiers in Public Health* 2019;**7**(14):141.

268. Haslam SA, Reicher SD, Platow M. *The New Psychology of Leadership*. London: Routledge 2020.

269. Haidt J. *The Righteous Mind: Why Good People Are Divided By Politics and Religion*. New York: Pantheon 2012.

270. Everett J, Colombatto C, Chituc C, et al. The effectiveness of moral messages on public health behavioral intentions during the COVID-19 pandemic. *PsyArXiv* 2020.

271. Shen L. Targeting smokers with empathy appeal antismoking public service announcements: A field experiment. *Journal of Health Communication* 2015;**20**:573–80. https://doi.org/101080/1081073020151012236.

272. Popper K. *The Logic of Scientific Discovery*. London: Routledge & Kegan Paul 1959.

273. Weiss CH. How can theory-based evaluation make greater headway? *Evaluation Review* 1997;**21**:501–24.

274. Davey C, Hassan S, Cartwright N, et al. *Designing Evaluations to Provide Evidence to Inform Action in New Settings*. London: Department for International Development 2019.

275. Carpenter K, Stoner S, Mikko A, et al. Efficacy of a web-based intervention to reduce sexual risk in men who have sex with men. *AIDS Behavior* 2010;**14**(3):549–57. https://doi.org/10.1007/s10461-009-9578-2.

276. Fisher J, Fisher W, Misovich S, et al. Changing AIDS risk behavior: Effects of an intervention emphasizing AIDS risk reduction information, motivation, and behavioral skills in a college student population. *Health Psychology Review* 1996;**15**:114–23.

277. Miller WR, Rollnick S. *Motivational Interviewing: Preparing People to Change*. New York: Guilford Press 2002.

278. Reback C, Fletcher J, Swendeman D, et al. Theory-based text-messaging to reduce methamphetamine use and HIV sexual risk behaviors among men who have sex with men: Automated unidirectional delivery outperforms bidirectional peer interactive delivery. *AIDS and Behavior* 2019;**23**(1):37–47. https://doi.org/10.1007/s10461-018-2225-z.

279. Bandura A. Social cognitive theory: An agentic perspective. *Annual Review of Psychology* 2001;**52**:1–26.

280. Becker MH. The health belief model: A decade later. *Health Education & Behavior* 1984;**11**(1):1–47. https://doi.org/101177/1090198111418108.

281. Melendez-Torres GJ, Meiksin R, Witzel TC, et al. eHealth interventions to address HIV and other sexually transmitted infections, sexual risk behavior, substance use, and mental ill-health in men who have sex with men: Systematic review and meta-analysis. *JMIR Public Health Surveillance* 2022;**8**(4):e27061.

282. Melendez-Torres GJ, Orr N, Farmer C, et al. School-based interventions To Prevent Dating and Relationship Violence and Gender-Based Violence (STOP-DRV-GBV): systematic review to understand characteristics, mechanisms, implementation and effectiveness. *Public Health Research* (in press).

283. Ponsford R, Falconer J, Melendez-Torres GJ, et al. Whole-school interventions promoting student commitment to school to prevent substance use and violence: Synthesis of theories of change. *Health Education (Online first)* 2022. https://doi.org/101177/00178969221100892.

284. Cross D, Barnes A, Cardoso P, et al. Cyber-friendly schools. In Campbell M, Bauman S, eds. *Reducing Cyberbullying in Schools: International Evidence-Based Best Practices*. Cambridge, MA: Academic Press 2018:95–108.

285. Bronfenbrenner U. *The Ecology of Human Development: Experiments by Nature and Design*. Cambridge, MA: Harvard University Press 1979.

286. Boudon R. What middle-range theories are. *Contemporary Sociology* 1991;**20**(4):519–22.

287. Iasuutari P. Theorizing in qualitative research: A cultural studies perspective. *Qualitative Inquiry* 1996;**2**(4):371–84.

288. Turner JH. Must sociological theory and sociological practice be so far apart? *Sociological Perspectives* 1998;**41**(2):243–58.

Index

Printed in the United States
by Baker & Taylor Publisher Services

Printed in the United States
by Baker & Taylor Publisher Services